Medical Terminology for Health Professions
3rd Edition

Instructor's Resource Kit

Compiled by
Ann Ehrlich

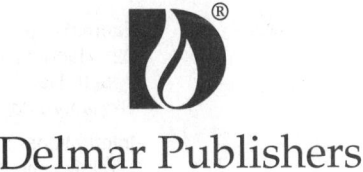

Delmar Publishers

I(T)P® International Thomson Publishing

Albany • Bonn • Boston • Cincinnati • Detroit • London • Madrid
Melbourne • Mexico City • New York • Pacific Grove • Paris • San Francisco
Singapore • Tokyo • Toronto • Washington

NOTICE TO THE READER

Publisher does not warrant or guarantee any of the products described herein or perform any independent analysis in connection with any of the product information contained herein. Publisher does not assume, and expressly disclaims, any obligation to obtain and include information other than that provided to it by the manufacturer.

The reader is expressly warned to consider and adopt all safety precautions that might be indicated by the activities described herein and to avoid all potential hazards. By following the instructions contained herein, the reader willingly assumes all risks in connection with such instructions.

The publisher makes no representations or warranties of any kind, including but not limited to, the warranties of fitness for particular purpose or merchantability, nor are any such representations implied with respect to the material set forth herein, and the publisher takes no responsibility with respect to such material. The publisher shall not be liable for any special, consequential, or exemplary damages resulting, in whole or in part, from the readers' use of, or reliance upon, this material.

COPYRIGHT © 1997
By Delmar Publishers
an International Thomson Publishing company

Delmar Publishers' Online Services
To access Delmar on the World Wide Web, point your browser to: http://www.delmar.com/delmar.html
To access through Gopher: gopher://gopher.delmar.com
(Delmar Online is part of "thomson.com", an Internet site with information on more than 30 publishers of the International Thomson Publishing organization.)

For more information on our products and services: email: info@delmar.com or call 800-347-7707

The ITP logo is a trademark under license

Printed in the United States of America

For information, contact:

Delmar Publishers
3 Columbia Circle, Box 15015
Albany, New York 12212-5015

International Thomson Publishing Europe
Berkshire House 168-173
High Holborn
London, WC1V7AA
England

Thomas Nelson Australia
102 Dodds Street
South Melbourne, 3205
Victoria, Australia

Nelson Canada
1120 Birchmont Road
Scarborough, Ontario
Canada M1K 5G4

International Thomson Editores
Campos Eliseos 385, Piso 7
Col Polanco
11560 Mexico D F Mexico

International Thomson Publishing GmbH
Königswinterer Strasse 418
53227 Bonn
Germany

International Thomson Publishing Asia
221 Henderson Road
#05-10 Henderson Building
Singapore 0315

International Thomson Publishing–Japan
Hirakawacho Kyowa Building, 3F
2-2-1 Hirakawacho
Chiyoda-ku, Tokyo 102
Japan

All rights reserved. The publisher grants that this work may be reproduced or used in any form, by any means—graphic, electronic, or mechanical, including photocopying, recording, taping, or information storage and retrieval systems—without written permission of the publisher when used in conjunction with *Medical Terminology for Health Professions*, 3E.

5 6 7 8 9 10 XXX 02 01 00 99 98

Library of Congress Card No: 96-4882
ISBN 0-8273-7843-2

Contents

Preface	ix
Contributors	ix
Reviewers	xii
How to Use this Resource Kit	xiii

SECTION A TIPS FOR NEW TEACHERS   1

Learning Styles 1
The Supportive Classroom 2
Teaching Medical Terminology as Competency-Based Education 3
Test Construction 5
Course Planning Suggestions 5

SECTION B TEACHING AIDS   10

Activity Cards 11
Audiotapes 11
Case Studies 12
Computer Teaching Aids 15
Crossword Puzzles 15
Current Medical Information Scrapbook 16
Flash Cards 16
Fill in the Blanks 17
Overhead Transparencies 18
Personal Experiences 18
Puzzling Pairs 19

Resource Files 20
Search and Report 21
Study Suggestions 21
Team and Class Activities 22
Videotapes 22
Visual Aids 22
Write-a-Story 23

SECTION C CLASSROOM ACTIVITIES   24

Aerobic Action 25
Alphabet Soup 26
Bingo 27
Body Planes and Directions 27
Bowl Games 28
Concentration 29
Create-a-Word 30
Definition Bee 30
Hangman 31
Human Word Building 32
Jeopardy!® 33
Labeling Body Parts 33
Medical Term Dissection 34
Medical Terminology Challenge 35
Random Access 36
Scrabble® 36
Speed Writing 37
Spelling Bee 37
Terminology Battle 39
Term or Definition? 39
Terminology Pursuit 40
The Living Heart 41
Twenty Questions 42
Understanding Afferent and Efferent Neurons 43
Watermelon Surgery 44

SECTION D MEDICAL WORD PART BINGO   45

Medical Word Part Bingo Caller's List 47
Medical Word Part Bingo Cards 48

SECTION E JEOPARDY!®   60

Grid for Medical Word Part Jeopardy! 62
Questions for Medical Word Part Jeopardy! 63

Grid for Body System Jeopardy! 65
Questions for Skeletal System Jeopardy! 66
Questions for Muscular System Jeopardy! 67
Questions for Cardiovascular System Jeopardy! 68
Questions for Respiratory System Jeopardy! 69
Questions for Digestive System Jeopardy! 70
Questions for Urinary System Jeopardy! 71
Questions for Nervous System Jeopardy! 72
Questions for Integumentary System Jeopardy! 73
Questions for Reproductive Systems Jeopardy! 74

SECTION F CROSSWORD PUZZLES — 76

Medical Word Part Crossword Puzzle 77
Medical Specialities Crossword Puzzle 78
The Skeletal System Crossword Puzzle 80
The Muscular System Crossword Puzzle 82
The Cardiovascular System Crossword Puzzle 84
The Respiratory System Crossword Puzzle 86
The Digestive System Crossword Puzzle 88
The Urinary System Crossword Puzzle 90
The Nervous System Crossword Puzzle 92
The Integumentary System Crossword Puzzle 94
The Reproductive Systems Crossword Puzzle 96
The General Medical Terminology Crossword Puzzle 98
Answers to Crossword Puzzles 100

SECTION G ACTIVITY CARDS — 103

Medical Specialty Activity Cards 105
The Skeletal System Activity Cards 109
The Muscular System Activity Cards 113
The Cardiovascular System Activity Cards 117
The Immune System and Oncology Activity Cards 121
The Respiratory System Activity Cards 123
The Digestive System Activity Cards 127
The Urinary System Activity Cards 131
The Nervous System Activity Cards 135
Eyes and Ears Activity Cards 139
The Integumentary System Activity Cards 141
The Endocrine System Activity Cards 145
The Male Reproductive System Activity Cards 147
Pregnancy and Childbirth Activity Cards 149
The Female Reproductive System Activity Cards 151
Examination Terminology Activity Cards 155
Endoscopic Examination Activity Cards 157
General Medical Terminology Activity Cards 159

SECTION H CASE STUDIES   163

Case 1 History and Physical Examination: Appendicitis,
    Operative Report and Discharge Summary........................... 165
Case 2 History and Physical Examination: Cardiology..................... 169
Case 3 Radiology Report: Chest 171
Case 4 Ultrasound Report: Prostate..................................... 172
Case 5 Case Summary: Ewing Sarcoma 173
Case 6 Case Summary: Diabetes/Hypertension 175
Case 7 Consultation Report: Ophthalmology 178
Case 8 Consultation Report: Allergy 179
Case 9 Consultation Report: ENT (Ears, Nose, Throat) 181
Case 10 Consultation Report: Hematology/Oncology 183
Case 11 Consultation Report: AIDS Patient 186
Case 12 Consultation Report: Ophthalmology 189
Case 13 Operative Report: Total Colonoscopy 191
Case 14 Operative Report: Cysto-scopy 193
Case 15 Operative Report: Open Reduction/Internal Fixation
    of Ulnar Fracture 195
Case 16 Operative Report: Cesarean Section 197
Case 17 Operative Report: Femoral Artery Bypass 199
Case 18 Operative Report: Kidney Tumor................................ 201
Case 19 Operative Report: Mastectomy 203
Case 20 Discharge Summary: Colostomy Closure 205
Case 21 Discharge Summary: Diverticulitis 206
Case 22 Discharge Summary: Fractured Spine 208
Case 23 Discharge Summary: Pneumonia 210
Case 24 Discharge Summary: Variety of Problems, Internal Medicine 212

SECTION I ART FOR OVERHEAD TRANSPARENCIES   214

Overview of Art for Overhead Transparencies 214
Medical Terminology Word Parts 215
Major Body Planes 216
The Skeleton (anterior view)... 217
The Skeleton (posterior view) 218
The Skeleton (lateral view) 219
The Skull (anterior view).. 220
The Skull (lateral view) 221
Major Muscles (anterior view)... 222
Major Muscles (posterior view) 223
The Heart (external view) 224
The Heart (cross section) 225
Systemic and Pulmonary Circulation 226
Structures of the Upper Respiratory Tree 227
Structures of the Bronchial Tree 228
Major Structures of the Digestive System 229
Major Structures of the Urinary System 230

A Nephron Unit and Related Structures 231
The Brain, Spinal Cord, and Spinal Nerves (posterior view) 232
The Brain (external lateral view) 233
The Brain (cross section) 234
The Eye (cross section) 235
The Ear (cross section) 236
Structures of the Skin (cross section) 237
Structures of the Endocrine System 238
The Male Pelvis (cross section) 239
The Female Pelvis (cross section) 240
The Developing Fetus (cross section) 241
Examination Positions 242

Preface

The previous edition of the *Instructor's Resource Kit* was created using ideas from more than 100 instructors, like you, who teach medical terminology in a variety of settings. These teachers are listed in the Contributors section and again we want to express a very special thank you to each one.

When planning this edition, we asked teachers who were using the previous edition to give us their feedback and suggestions as to how it could be improved. We have incorporated their recommendations and ideas to make this edition even more useful. This includes adding a new section, improving the organization of the other sections, and including as many activities as possible that are ready to use. This new organization is explained under the heading of *How to Use this Resource Kit*.

Working on this project is a particular joy for me because it provides unique interaction with teachers and allows all of us to tap into their creativity. These are ideas that have been used by successful teachers. If they are new to you, I think you and your students will enjoy them too. I want to use this opportunity to thank everyone who shared so unselfishly to make this a valuable resource for all teachers of medical terminology.

Ann Ehrlich

CONTRIBUTORS

Irma Aguilar, Odessa College, Odessa, TX.

Karen Bargell, Northeastern Junior College, Sterling, CO.

Judith Bastin, MS, RT, Director Radiation Therapy Program, National-Louis University, Evanston, IL.

Deborah K. Bauert, MS, RTR, Casper College, Casper WY.

Brenda J. Beasley, RN, BS, EMT-Paramedic, EMS Program Director, Southern Union State Junior College, EMS Program, Wadley, AL.

Dr. Mary Jo Belenski, Montclair State College, Upper Montclair, NJ.

Linda Berry, RN, MSN, Nursing Instructor, Front Range Community College, Fort Collins, CO.

Lynn Blom, National College, Rapid City, SC.

Carrie Boatman, CMT, Instructor, Medical Transcription Program, Sacramento County Office of Education, Sacramento, CA.

Pamela Borrelli, RN, MN, CCRN, Adjunct Instructor, College of the Canyons, Valencia, CA.

ix

Phyllis J. Broughton, Pitt Community College, Greenville, NC.

Sue Buboltz, Madison Area Technical College, Madison, WI.

Rufus Butler, Delta Schools, Lafayette, LA.

Kathy J. Caballero, Program Director and MA Instructor, American Institute of Technology, Phoenix, AZ.

Toni Cade, RRA, MDB, Medical Record Administration, University of Southwestern Louisiana, Lafayette, LA.

Thomas Carey, Berkshire Community College, Pittsfield, MA.

Adrienne L. Carter-Ward, CMA-RMA, National Education Center, San Bernardino Super School, San Bernardino, CA.

Carol Cassell, RN, Associate Faculty, Butte Community College, Oroville, CA.

Jeanne M. Clerc, EdD MT(ASCP), SH, Eastern Michigan University, Ypsilanti, MI.

Kathy Collier, Foster Meade Avec.

Betty M. Cooper, AA, Instructor, Lakeland-Medical Dental Academy, Minneapolis, MN.

Charles R. Crew, Oklahoma Junior College, Tulsa, OK.

Martha Crisp, Owensboro Campus, Kentucky Technical School, Owensboro, KY.

Carol Crum, Marion Technical College.

Thor Dekker, Pacific Coast College, Chula Vista, CA.

Sandra Denton, MA, Career City College, Gainesville, FL.

David E. Ehrhardt, RN, BSN, BAed, CCRN, PHN, National Education Center, Oakland, CA.

Margaret Eldridge, RN, MHED, Allied Health Department, Butte Community College, Chico, CA.

Nancy Enck, MD, BSN, RN, CMA, Division of Allied Health Technology, The University of Akron, Akron OH.

Donna J. Endicott, Xavier University.

Patricia Etryre-Zacher, Northern Illinois University, DeKalb, IL.

Joyce Garibay, Medical Office Assistant Program Coordinator/Instructor, Lane Community College, Eugene OR.

Joanne Glaser, West Virginia Career College, Charleston, WV.

Gary S. Green, Berkeley Adult School, Berkeley, CA.

Jo Grove, RN, St. Louis Community College at Forest Park, St. Louis, MO.

Judy Gust, MEd, Medical Office Instructor, Rochester Community College, Rochester, MN.

Rebecca Hageman, Hutchinson Community College, Hutchinson, KS.

Prof. Emmajane P. Hagenbuch, BS, MEd, Office Administration Department, Northampton Community College, Bethlehem, PA.

Dona Halbert, BS, Instructor-Medical Office Management, Tyler Junior College, Tyler, TX.

Marilyn Hamilton, Pueblo College of Business and Technology, Pueblo, CO.

Brenda Haueisen, Westshore Community College Tec Prep, Scottville, MI.

Sharolyn Heatwole, RN, MSN, J. Sargeant Reynolds Community College, Richmond VA.

Kathleen Hess, RNBS, Antonelli Medical and Professional Institute, Pottstown, PA.

Crystal Higgins, Southeast Community College, Beatrice, NE.

Jane A. Hlopko, MA, ART, Assistant Professor, MRT Program Broome Community College, Binghamton, NY.

Joyce C. Houea, RN, Front Range Community College, Fort Collins, CO.

Dr. Mamie R. Howard, Mott Community College, Flint, MI.

Cathy D. Hunt, Henderson Community College, Henderson, KY.

Charlotte A. Jensen, Cabrillo College.

Peggy Kerr, MS, PT, Director of PTA Program, Genesee Community College, Batavia, NY.

A. Kiernan, Briarwood College.

Susan Kilburn, Crawford County Area Vo-Tech, Meadville, PA.

Peggy Knittel, MD, Eastern Wyoming College, Torrington, WY.

Cindy Konrad, MS, RN, Ferris State University, Big Rapids, MI.

Mary Jane Koranda, BSN, RN, Department of Nursing, Dodge City Community College, Dodge City, KA.

Maria Krebsbach, Southern Technical College, Shreveport, LA.

Dennis Leaver, Southern Maine Technical College, South Portland, ME.

Martha R. Leonard, BA, MA, MPH, Midlands Technical College, Columbia, SC.

Cathy Lipot, ROP/Santa Ana Unified School District, Santa Ana, CA.

Sharon Lynn, MTI Business College, Sacramento, CA.

Debbie Marcy, NCCC, Saranac Lake, NY.

Karen Melcher, RRA, Northeast Iowa Community College, Calmar, IA.

Melinda D. Montavon, COTA/L, Instructor, OTA program, Shawnee State University, Portsmouth, OH.

Lou Ann Mozinjo, Farmville Central High School, Farmville, NC.

Reggie Murray, Community High School, Fort Keat, ME.

Phyllis Parks, CMA, AC, Olympic College, Bremerton, WA.

Elaine O. Patrikas, MA, RRA, Professor, Department of Health Records Administration, Temple University, Philadelphia, PA.

A. Christine Payne, RN, MA, Sarasota County Technical Institute, Sarasota, FL.

Dan Points, Dean, Health Sciences Division, Rose State College, Midwest City, OK.

Dee Poston, Shawnee Community College, Ullin, IL.

Vicki Prater, Concorde Career College, San Bernardino, CA.

Dr. LaVerne Ramacker, Indiana University Northwest, Gary, IN.

Virginia R. Reiser, Leslie County Vocational School. Hyden, KY.

Elaine Rejimbal, Lake Sumter Community College, Leesburg, FL.

Sondra Richards, MS, RT(R), Program Director, Radiological Technology, Kilgore College, Kilgore, TX.

Jaretta Roeoff, Indiana Vocational Technical College, Terre Haute, IN.

Theodore R. Salaiz, Surgical Tecnhology, Community College of Denver, Denver Co.

Mary Jo Schleif, RN CHUC, Hennepin Technical College, Brooklyn Park, MN.

Donna L. Shea, NEC Skadrow Campus, San Bernardino, CA.

B.J. Smith, Canterbury Career School, Renaissance, NY.

Mary Spivey, Broward Community College, Davie, FL.

Saundra Stevens, RN, BSN, CMA, Coordinator, Medical Assisting Program, Southern State Community College, Hillsboro, OH.

Marliss Strange, University of Oregon, Eugene, OR.

Mr. Stringer, Baton Rouge Vo-Tech Institute.

Cynthia Swann, Concorde Career Institute, Denver CO.

Francine Tabana-Belin, Borough of Manhattan Community College, New York, NY.

Mary Ann Talley, BSN, MPA, EMT, Director, Center for Emergency Response Training, Division of EMS Education, University of South Alabama, Mobile, AL.

Shirley J. Tangredi-Dye, BS, RN, CMA-C, Bryant and Stratton Business Institute, Rochester, NY.

Sheila Teman, Hillcrest High School, Jamacia NY.

Nancy Thomas, Mount Marty College, Yankton, SD.

Donna R. Townsend, Renton Technical College, Renton, WA.

Patty Vail, RN, MA, Director Vocational Nurse and Psychiatric Technician Programs, Napa Valley College, Napa, CA.

Dee Vandercook, Allan Hancock College, Santa Maria CA.

Linda E. Villejas, LVN, CMA, Career Centers of Texas-El Paso Inc.

Winfred E. Watkins, McLennan Community College, Waco, TX.

Margaret Watson, NSSBS, Londonbry, NH.

Brenda S. Webster-Houch, Northern Tier Career Center.

Sara Wellman, ART, School of Allied Health Sciences, Indiana University Northwest, Gary, IN.

Dianne M Whalen, MT(ASCP), CMA-C, Northwestern Michigan College, Traverse City, MI.

Herbert E. Wheeler, Hartford Area Vocational Center, White River Junction, CT.

Reviewers

Barbara Brown, MEd, BSN, RN, Robeson Community College, Lumberton, SC

Eudelia Thomas, MS, RRA, Florida Community College, Jacksonville, FL

Connie Dempsey, RN, BSN, MSN, Stark Technical College, Canton, OH

Donna Shea, CRT, RMA, CMA-AC, RPT, CPT, CSI Skadrow, San Bernandino, CA

Iristine Graham, LPN, Specializing in You (Staff Development), Blue Springs, MO

Jean Hale, Glenville, NY

How to Use this Resource Kit

Whenever possible the ideas and activities in this kit are ready to use or require only minimal preparation. In keeping with this, you are welcome to duplicate any of these materials for use in your classroom. For your convenience, this *Instructor's Resource Kit* is organized into nine sections:

1. **Section A: Tips for New Teachers.** This section covers Learning Styles, The Supportive Classroom, Teaching Medical Terminology as Competency-Based Education, Test Construction, and Course Planning Suggestions.

2. **Section B: Teaching Aids.** This section includes 18 ideas for teaching aids that you can use in the your classroom. To help you review these quickly, an "Overview of Teaching Aids" appears at the beginning of the section.

3. **Section C: Class Activities.** This section includes 25 activities for class, team, and small group use to make practice sessions more effective and more fun. To help you find appropriate activities quickly, an "Overview of Classroom Activities" appears at the beginning of the section.

4. **Section D: Medical Word Part Bingo.** This is a complete Bingo game that is ready to photocopy and play. It includes a caller's list and 10 different Bingo cards to accompany the list.

5. **Section E: Jeopardy!™** Jeopardy!™ is such a popular classroom activity that this section includes (1) a ready-to-copy-and-use "Medical Word Part Jeopardy!™ game, (2) plus nine ready-to-copy-and-use "Body System Jeopardy!™ games. There are also additional forms to help you develop your own Jeopardy!™ questions.

6. **Section F: Crossword Puzzles and Solutions.** This section includes 12 crossword puzzles covering the major body systems. Each puzzle contains between 30 to 40 medical terms that should be challenging to your students.

7. **Section G: Activity Cards.** This section contains 18 sets of activity cards. These are arranged like flash cards with the term on the front and the definition on

the back. These may be copied, then separated for use as needed with many of the classroom activities.

8. **Section H: Case Studies.** At the beginning of this section there is an overview of the 24 case studies. Also, there are five case study questions included at the end of each case. These are excellent for student review and as class discussion questions. As an additional aid, included in Section B as part of the discussion of the uses of case studies, Figure 4 lists the "Case Studies by Body Systems."

9. **Section I: Art for Overhead Transparencies.** This section contains 28 pieces of art that can be used to create overhead transparencies or may be duplicated for other classroom uses.

SECTION A

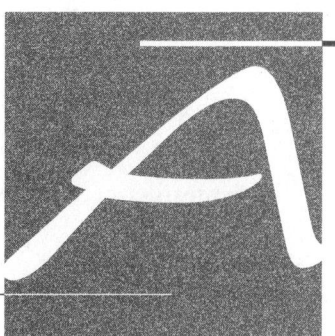

Tips for New Teachers

This section contains information and ideas of particular interest to a beginning teacher (such as a health care professional who is just starting to teach), an instructor who has never taught medical terminology before, and an experienced teacher who is looking for new insights. The topics discussed here include:

- Learning Styles
- The Supportive Classroom
- Teaching Medical Terminology as Competency-Based Education
- Test Construction
- Course Planning Suggestions

LEARNING STYLES

Educational theorists describe students as having four distinct learning styles or orientations. Although presented as distinct orientations, it is important to recognize that most students actually learn through a combination of these four styles: reading, visual, auditory, and kinesthetic.

Reading. Reading learners remember best those things they have read and they do well with textbook assignments and studying the topic on a printed page.

Visual. Visual learners want to see it happen! Visually oriented class presentations such as diagrams, overhead transparencies, demonstrations, and videotapes are helpful to these (and all of your students).

Auditory. Auditory learners remember best those things they have heard as in a class presentation or on an audiotape—assuming these were interesting enough to hold their attention.

Audiotapes are important in helping all students learn to pronounce medical terms properly and the discussion of audiotapes in the "Teaching Aids Section" contains suggestions on how to fully involve students in listening and working with these tapes.

Kinesthetic. Kinesthetic learners remember best those things they actually experience, for example, performing muscle movements as they study the related terms. The needs of these students are more difficult to accommodate. However, to help you these kinesthetic activities are included in this resource kit: Aerobic Action, The Living Heart, and Understanding Afferent and Efferent Neurons.

Involving All the Senses

Although these classifications are recent, the concept is not really new. The Chinese proverb *"I hear and I forget, I see and I remember, I do and I understand"* clearly demonstrates that the least learning occurs when students passively sit and listen to a lecture.

Your goal in class planning should be to have students actively participate and to fully involve as many of the senses as possible. This teaching format accommodates differing learning styles, aids in holding the student's attention, and makes the class much more interesting for both the students and teacher.

Verbal and Visual Feedback

Generous use of the board during class helps students because they both hear and see what is being discussed. Also, when students answer questions everyone receives more feedback if the answer is given verbally and then written on the board. You can write the correct answer as it is given or you can have the student write the answer. Because this may be threatening to some students, you can use this as an opportunity to praise a correct answer.

Using multiple colors on the board also helps students remember better or to clarify concepts. As an example, when teaching the concept of word parts, use one color for prefixes, another for combining forms, and a third color for suffixes.

The advance preparation for some of the classroom activities in Section C requires terms to be written on the board. An important reason for doing this is to have students hear, see, and experience the terms.

THE SUPPORTIVE CLASSROOM

Students who are comfortable in their surroundings do better in their studies, and an important factor in student success is their perception of a supportive environment in your classroom. In this setting students should feel free to learn without fear of ridicule or teasing. The manner in which you structure class activities helps to create such a setting.

Teams

The use of team activities in a class gets mixed reviews from experienced teachers. Those who are opposed to teams say that team formation divides the class, exposes students to being the last one selected, and may leave some team members doing all the work while others slide by.

Those who favor teams point out that health care workers usually work as part of a team. Therefore, learning to be good team players is a valuable skill. Certainly when a team is working at its best, the members help each other.

Some teachers establish teams that stay together throughout the course. These teams appoint a captain and are encouraged to adopt a team name. These teachers found that competition between teams improved student motivation. Such teams would be excellent for activities such as "Bowl Games" that are played throughout the course. Other teachers select teams randomly and use different teams for each activity. This gives the students experience in working with others they might not get to know as well.

Individual Responses

Many class activities require students to reply individually, and some students are really uncomfortable doing this. However, in a supportive atmosphere they can become more confident in their own abilities. You are an important role model in being supportive and not permitting sarcastic remarks when the student does not know the answer or gets it wrong.

Each-One-Teach-One

Peer teaching, in which students tutor each other, is a great way to help students learn and build self-confidence. As an example, if one student is having difficulty grasping the concept of medical word parts, another student can provide special help. Potentially, both students can benefit from the experience.

Memory Aids

Some of the most successful teachers of medical terminology have developed mnemonics (memory aids) to help their students remember difficult information. This is a great place to use your sense of humor. Often the silliest ones are the most effective, so do not be afraid to use them!

TEACHING MEDICAL TERMINOLOGY AS COMPETENCY-BASED EDUCATION

Competency-based education (CBE) is an exciting concept in that it states exactly which skills and behaviors the student is expected to have mastered on completion of the course. Although this concept is usually applied to clinical courses, it is also valid in teaching medical terminology.

In the language of CBE, **foundation knowledge** is the background information the student must have to achieve competency. A **competency** is the end result, i.e., the skill the student has mastered, and **evaluation criteria** are the conditions under which the student will demonstrate this mastery.

Foundation Knowledge

In a medical terminology course, the student must master the following foundation knowledge:

- Describe the three types of medical word parts and state how each type is used.
- Spell and define commonly used medical word parts.
- State the rules for the use of the combining vowel in medical terminology.
- Demonstrate the use of a medical dictionary in finding and defining medical terms.
- Describe the major body systems, their organs, and functions.

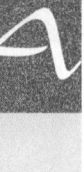

Competencies

In a medical terminology course, the student is expected to master these competencies:

- Pronounce, spell, and define commonly used medical terms relating to the pathology and procedures of the major body systems.
- Given the definition of a medical term made up of medical word parts, find the term and then spell and pronounce it correctly.
- Use a medical dictionary and similar reference materials to find the meaning of medical terms and commonly used abbreviations.

Evaluation Criteria

To evaluate competency in medical terminology, take into consideration the method of evaluation, whether or not the use of a medical dictionary is permitted, the time to be allowed to take the test, the passing score, and the number of attempts permitted.

Methods of Evaluation

A written test is the most efficient way of evaluating medical terminology competencies in a class setting. Almost any type of question can be used in the test. (See Test Construction, on page 5.)

To test spelling, you could include a brief dictation section at the beginning of the test. Then students are allowed to proceed through the rest at their own pace.

A written test does not evaluate the pronunciation of terms. If time permits, you could test students on this by taking them aside individually and listening to each pronounce a list of about 10 terms.

Use of a Medical Dictionary

Because the ability to use a medical dictionary is one of the competencies being tested, you will want to include questions to evaluate this skill.

Some teachers do not favor permitting dictionary use because they fear students will not study if they know they can look up answers. However, because looking terms up takes time and the student has limited time to complete the test, this is a limited advantage.

If you seriously oppose the use of a dictionary, include questions that test its use. As an example, *"What dictionary heading would you look under to find 'Sudden Infant Death Syndrome'?"*

Time Limit

A time limit is particularly important if students are allowed to use a medical dictionary. You determine how much time is allowed to take the test, which in part depends on the number of items in the test. The students should be informed about the time limit before the test session.

Passing Score

From the patient's point of view, only 100% performance by a health care worker is acceptable. However, in an academic setting the level of a passing score is usually determined by school policy.

Number of Attempts Permitted

Some teachers permit only one attempt at demonstrating a competency. This relates to the theory that in the workplace, there is only one opportunity to get it right.

Other teachers believe that students increase in competency each time they are evaluated; therefore if a student wants to improve a grade, a retest should be allowed. However, usually a 10-point penalty is assessed for each retest. This means that even if the student answered all the questions right on a retest, the highest score possible would be 90.

TEST CONSTRUCTION

The first step in test construction is not writing questions or gathering them from an electronic test bank. You should start by reviewing your course goals and determining exactly what you are testing for.

Because the skills being tested in a medical terminology course are cognitive, most written question formats are acceptable for testing. The primary exception to this is the use of true/false or other questions with only two answer choices that automatically give the student a 50–50 chance of guessing right.

Fill-In the blank questions are effective for testing the ability to read a definition and supply the term. Students need to understand in advance that the answer is not correct unless the term is spelled properly. The disadvantage is that these questions take longer to correct and computer scoring is not a possibility.

Labeling questions are most frequently used for anatomy and physiology questions. When using this type of question, be certain that the illustration is free of distractions and that the parts being questioned are clear.

Matching questions are particularly effective when a series of similar items are challenging to differentiate. As an example, types of muscle movements are well suited for a good matching question.

Multiple-Choice questions can be adapted to most topics and testing situations. For help in constructing these questions, see Figure 1 "Tips For Writing Multiple-Choice Questions."

COURSE PLANNING SUGGESTIONS

Developing the Syllabus

The preparation of a syllabus is the beginning point and an important part of your planning process. It is here that you determine what is to be taught, when it will be taught, and the method of presentation. When you are responsible for planning courses to be taught by several instructors, a well stated syllabus and course outline help to ensure that all class sections cover the same information. Figure 2 is a sample 16-week course syllabus based on the use of Ehrlich's *Medical Terminology for Health Professionals*, 3rd ed.

Planning the Course Outline

The course outline details what is to be covered during each week of the course. It also states the assignments students are expected to complete in preparation for class,

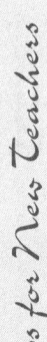

Tips for Writing Multiple-Choice Questions

The Stem

- The **stem** is an introductory question or incomplete statement to which the student must respond. The stem should be as short and simple as possible. You are testing the student's comprehension, not his or her ability to decipher complex questions.
- **Direct question.** A direct question stem, such as, *"Which medical term means vomiting blood?"* is the most effective format.
- **Incomplete sentence.** An incomplete sentence such as *"Vomiting blood is called"* is also effective.
- **Fill-In The Blank.** If the stem cannot be worded as a direct question or incomplete sentence, a fill-in the blank sentence is an acceptable alternative. As an example, *"Hematemesis means _____ blood."*
- A **negatively worded question**, such as *"Which of the following does not mean vomiting blood?"* is much more difficult because the student must first interpret the question and then find the answer.

The Choices

- The **choices** are one **correct answer** and the **distractors** (incorrect answers). An effective multiple-choice question has 4 possible answers. Fewer choices allow the student to guess more easily. More choices increase the difficulty of the question.
- If the stem is written as an incomplete sentence, the answers must flow to complete the sentence. Also, final punctuation for the sentence is placed after each answer.
- All distractors should be believable and fit with the question format.
- All answers should be of approximately equal length.
- Keep the answers as short as possible. Any term or phrase that appears in all of the answers probably should be moved to the stem.
- Avoid verbal similarities in wording the stem and the correct answer. This type of wording may provide a clue to the student.
- Arrange the answers in alphabetical or logical order such as from shortest to longest answer.

Figure 1

identifies when tests are scheduled, and helps to ensure that all class sections cover the same information. Figure 3 is a sample 16-week course outline based on the use of Ehrlich's *Medical Terminology for Health Professionals*, 3rd ed.

Each student should receive a copy of both the syllabus and course outline at the beginning of the course. This informs students exactly what is expected of them, and when, throughout the semester. This leaves no surprises, and no excuses. If students are taking this as a self-instructional course, these documents act as a guide through their studies.

Verifying the Course Description

Before starting to plan, read the description of your course as it appears in the school catalogue. If you have questions about it, ask your supervisor to be certain that this is an accurate description of what is to be taught. If you find discrepancies, they should be resolved before you plan your course.

Sample Syllabus for a 16-Week Medical Terminology Course

Course Name and Number: _____

Course Goal Statement: _____

Faculty Name(s) and Office Location(s): _____

Course Location: _____

Times and Day(s) Course Meets: _____

Attendance Policy: _____

Required Text(s):
   Ehrlich, Medical Terminology for Health Professions, 3rd ed.
   Optional: Audiotapes to accompany text.
   Optional: Student Practice Disk to accompany text.

Teaching Methods
   Chapter reading and exercise assignments are to be completed **before** class.
   Class time will be devoted to discussing content, presentation of enrichment materials, and the reinforcement required to master the topic.

Quizzes and Examinations:
   Chapter Quizzes: There <u>may be</u> a 25-question quiz at any class session.
   These <u>will not</u> be announced in advance.
   Word Part Test: There will be a test at the end of week 2.
   This will cover the word parts from Chapters 1 and 2.
   Mid-Term Examination: The mid-term examination will be given at the end of week 8.
   This test covers Chapters 1 through 7.
   Final Examination: The final examination will be given as scheduled during exam week.
   This test covers all course contents.

Evaluation Methods:
   1/3 of grade   Chapter exercises, class quizzes, attendance, and class participation.
   1/3 of grade   Mid-Term examination.
   1/3 of grade   Final examination.

Figure 2

Writing the Course Goal Statement

The first step in planning is to write a clearly phrased course goal statement. As an example, *"Upon completion of this course the student will be able to identify, spell, and define medical terms related to the diagnosis, pathology, and treatment of the major body systems."*

The development of this statement will clarify your thinking about the course. Later, this statement will make students aware of exactly what they are expected to learn in the course.

Identifying the Time Factors

Study the school calendar and determine how many weeks the course will run. During these weeks, how many actual class sessions are scheduled? Based on these calculations, you know how much time you have for presenting class work.

Sample Course Outline for a 16-Week Medical Terminology Course

WEEK 1   **Chapter 1 - Introduction to Medical Terminology**
Assignment: Study Chapter 1 and complete the exercises.
Optional: Listen to audiotape to accompany Chapter 1.
Student Practice Disk: Chapter 1 Exercises, Fun and Games.

WEEK 2   **Chapter 2 - Structure of the Human Body**
Assignment: Study Chapter 2 and complete the exercises.
Optional: Listen to audiotape to accompany Chapter 2
Student Practice Disk: Chapter 2 Exercises, Fun and Games.
Optional: Word Part Review exercises.
*** Word Part Test ***

WEEK 3   **Chapter 3 - The Skeletal System**
Assignment: Study Chapter 3 and complete the exercises.
Optional: Listen to audiotape to accompany Chapter 3.
Student Practice Disk: Chapter 3 Exercises, Fun and Games.

WEEK 4   **Chapter 4 - The Muscular System**
Assignment: Study Chapter 4 and complete the exercises.
Optional: Listen to audiotape to accompany Chapter 4.
Student Practice Disk: Chapter 4 Exercises, Fun and Games.

WEEK 5   **Chapter 5 - The Cardiovascular System**
Assignment: Study Chapter 5 and complete the exercises.
Optional: Listen to audiotape to accompany Chapter 5.
Student Practice Disk: Chapter 5 Exercises, Fun and Games.

WEEK 6   **Chapter 6 - The Lymphatic and Immune Systems**
Assignment: Study Chapter 6 and complete the exercises.
Optional: Listen to audiotape to accompany Chapter 6.
Student Practice Disk: Chapter 6 Exercises, Fun and Games.

WEEK 7   **Chapter 7 - The Respiratory System**
Assignment: Study Chapter 7 and complete the exercises.
Optional: Listen to audiotape to accompany Chapter 7.
Student Practice Disk: Chapter 7 Exercises, Fun and Games.

WEEK 8   *Assignment:* Complete classwork to date.
Review for mid-term examination.
*** Mid-Term Examination ***

WEEK 9   **Chapter 8 - The Digestive System**
Assignment: Study Chapter 8 and complete the exercises.
Optional: Listen to audiotape to accompany Chapter 8.
Student Practice Disk: Chapter 8 Exercises, Fun and Games.

WEEK 10   **Chapter 9 - The Urinary System**
Assignment: Study Chapter 9 and complete the exercises.
Optional: Listen to audiotape to accompany Chapter 9.
Student Practice Disk: Chapter 9 Exercises, Fun and Games.

WEEK 11   **Chapter 10 - The Nervous System**
Assignment: Study Chapter 10 and complete the exercises.
Optional: Listen to audiotape to accompany Chapter 10.
Student Practice Disk: Chapter 10 Exercises, Fun and Games.
(continued)

Figure 3

	Chapter 11 - The Special Senses
	Assignment: Study Chapter 11 and complete the exercises.
	Optional: Listen to audiotape to accompany Chapter 11.
	Student Practice Disk: Chapter 11 Exercises, Fun and Games.
WEEK 12	**Chapter 12 - The Integumentary System**
	Assignment: Study Chapter 12 and complete the exercises.
	Optional: Listen to audiotape to accompany Chapter 12.
	Student Practice Disk: Chapter 12 Exercises, Fun and Games.
	Chapter 13 - The Endocrine System
	Assignment: Study Chapter 13 and complete the exercises.
	Optional: Listen to audiotape to accompany Chapter 13.
	Student Practice Disk: Chapter 13 Exercises, Fun and Games.
WEEK 13	**Chapter 14 - The Reproductive Systems**
	Assignment: Study Chapter 14 and complete the exercises.
	Optional: Listen to audiotape to accompany Chapter 14.
	Student Practice Disk: Chapter 14 Exercises, Fun and Games.
WEEK 14	**Chapter 15 - Diagnostic and Imaging Procedures**
	Assignment: Study Chapter 15 and complete the exercises.
	Optional: Listen to audiotape to accompany Chapter 15.
	Student Practice Disk: Chapter 15 Exercises, Fun and Games.
	Chapter 16 - Pharmacology and General Medical Terminology
	Assignment: Study Chapter 16 and complete the exercises.
	Optional: Listen to audiotape to accompany Chapter 16.
	Student Practice Disk: Chapter 16 Exercises, Fun and Games.
WEEK 15	*Assignment:* Complete remaining classwork.
	Review for the final examination.
WEEK 16	*** Final Examination ***

Figure 3 (*continued*)

Establishing Priorities

If you have a 16-week course, and a 16-chapter textbook, planning is relatively easy, i.e., present one chapter per week. If you do not have this much class time, then you must prioritize and determine which topics and body systems are of the greatest importance to your students.

All medical terminology students need to start by learning about word parts. After they have mastered this, they are ready to progress to the study of specific body systems. The priorities you have established determine which systems are most important and should be studied first.

Class Planning

You will want to expand your copy to include session-by-session planning so you can have visual aids and activities in preparation for each class.

This resource kit is designed to help with that planning. You will want to take advantage of the information concerning 18 Teaching Aids and 25 Classroom Activities plus the resources to be used with them.

SECTION B

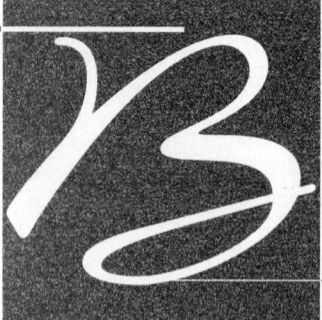

Teaching Aids

Overview of Teaching Aids

1. **Activity Cards**—Suggestions for the use of the cards found in Section G.
2. **Audiotapes**—Suggestions of ways to create and use audiotapes in the classroom or by students working on their own.
3. **Case Studies**—Suggestions on how to use the case studies found in Section H.
4. **Computer Teaching Aids**—Suggestions and listings of some of the most exciting new developments in the use of computerized aids for teaching medical terminology.
5. **Crossword Puzzles**—Suggestions on how to use the crossword puzzles found in Section F.
6. **Current Medical Information Scrapbook**—Suggestions on how to create and use this valuable classroom resource.
7. **Flash Cards**—Suggestions on how to create and use flash cards.
8. **Fill In The Blanks**—Suggestions on how to create and use fill-in the blank activities in the classroom. Includes a sample story.
9. **Overhead Transparencies**—Suggested uses of the art for overhead transparencies found in Section I.
10. **Personal Experiences**—Suggested uses of other people's personal experiences to help students recognize that the medical terminology they are learning is essential to their success in the health care career of their choice.
11. **Puzzling Pairs**—A suggestion to help students master the "puzzling pairs" of medical terms that sound alike and/or are contrasting in meaning.
12. **Resource Files**—Suggestions on how to establish and use this valuable teaching resource.
13. **Search And Report**—A suggested assignment that provides students with experience in seeking out information and provides enrichment materials for the entire class.
14. **Study Suggestions**—Ideas that may help your students learn study habits that will make learning medical terminology easier.

15. **Team And Class Activities**—A listing that will help you select activities suited for different types of class room situations.
16. **Videotapes**—Suggested uses and sources of videotapes.
17. **Visual Aids**—Suggested uses and sources of visual aids for classroom use.
18. **Write-A-Story**—A suggested written class assignment that is an interesting way to have students work with the terms they are learning.

ACTIVITY CARDS

Many of the activities in this resource kit call for the use of slips of paper containing a medical term or a definition. Section G features 18 sets of activities cards that may be copied to fill this need.

Suggestions

- You are welcome to copy these cards for use with activities found in Section C.
- For ease of use, the cards are organized by body system.
- Also use them like flash cards for medical term review in which the student must supply either the term or the definition.

Note: The "sounds like" pronunciation on these cards is reprinted, with permission, from Ehrlich's *Medical Terminology For Health Professions*, 3rd ed, Delmar Publishers, Albany, NY 1997.

AUDIOTAPES

Audiotapes are a versatile teaching aid for use in the classroom or by students working on their own.

Suggestions

- **Tapes to Accompany the Text.** If these are available, use them to help students learn how to pronounce new medical terms and to reinforce the definition of each term.
- **Word Lists.** If there is a word list in the text to accompany the tape, students should follow this and check each term as it is pronounced. This actively involves the students in the process and improves their concentration.
- **Using Audiotapes in Class.** Some teachers like to use the tape at the beginning of the class period to get the students "warmed up." Other teachers use the tape at the end of the class to reinforce the material presented in class.
- **Student Copies of Audiotapes.** When students have their own copies of the audiotapes they can review even while driving or jogging. This allows students to use the tape when and as often as they wish.

Additional Suggestions

- **Spelling Tests.** Some teachers like to use audiotapes to provide the terms for a spelling test.

- **Transcription Exercises.** In classes when students are also learning transcription, audiotapes can be used as beginning transcription exercises.

Case Study Audiotapes

You are welcome to create audiotapes of the case studies found in Section H. These may be used for listening practice and as transcription exercises. Beginning students will find these tapes most helpful if they have a printed copy of the report to follow as they listen to the tape.

If you are creating tapes for transcription exercises, you may want to use several voices including some foreign accents.

Tapes of Lectures

Another interesting idea is to encourage students to tape your lectures. Then the students can go back over these lectures as many times as needed to master the material.

There are times when a student really <u>must</u> miss a lecture. To help students overcome this problem, some teachers tape each lecture. These audiotapes are duplicated and available for sign-out to a student who is really motivated and wants to catch up.

CASE STUDIES

Case studies are a valuable resource because they clearly demonstrate how terms the student is learning in the classroom are applied in the real world. Section H includes 24 case studies prepared by Benna Kisin, Certified Medical Transcriptionist (CMT). These are based on actual reports from a variety of medical specialties with only the names changed to protect the privacy of the patient and physician. You are welcome to duplicate them for class use.

For ease of use, Section H also includes a short description of each case study. Figure 4 shows the cases organized by applicable body systems.

Case Studies by Body System

Case Number and Type of Report		Comments
Introduction to Case Studies		
Case 1	History and Physical Examination, Operative Report, and Discharge Summary.	Three reports follow a patient through the diagnosis and treatment of appendicitis.
The Skeletal System		
Case 5	Case Summary	Ongoing treatment for Ewing's sarcoma
Case 15	Operative Report	Open reduction of a fracture
Case 10	Consultation Report	Rheumatoid arthritis
Case 22	Discharge Summary	Multiple compression fractures
The Cardiovascular System		
Case 2	History and Physical Examination	Possible congestive heart failure
	(continued)	

Figure 4

Case Number and Type of Report		Comments
The Cardiovascular System (continued)		
Case 6	Case Summary	Congestive heart failure and hypertension
Case 10	Consultation Report	Anemia
Case 17	Operative Report	Femoral artery bypass
Case 24	Discharge Summary	Ventricular tachycardia
Lymphatic and Immune Lymphatic Systems (including Oncology)		
Case 5	Case Summary	Ongoing treatment for Ewing's sarcoma
Case 8	Consultation Report	Allergies
Case 10	Consultation Report	Possible autoimmune disease
Case 11	Consultation Report	Ongoing consultation for patient with AIDS
Case 18	Operative Report	Removal of Wilms' tumor of the left kidney
Case 19	Operative Report	Modified radical mastectomy
The Respiratory System		
Case 3	Radiology Report	Chest x-ray
Case 23	Discharge Summary	Pneumonia
The Digestive System		
Case 1	History and Physical Examination, Operative Report, and Discharge Summary.	Appendicitis
Case 10	Consultation Report	Recurrent partial bowel obstruction
Case 13	Operative Report	Total colonoscopy
Case 20	Discharge Summary	Colostomy closure
Case 21	Discharge Summary	Sigmoid diverticulitis
The Urinary System		
Case 6	Case Summary	Renal failure
Case 14	Operative Report	Cystoscopy
Case 18	Operative Report	Removal of Wilms' tumor of the left kidney
The Nervous System and Special Senses		
Case 7	Consultation Report	Eye infection
Case 9	Consultation report	Paroxysmal positional vertigo (dizziness)
Case 12	Consultation Report	Cataract surgery and follow-up care
The Endocrine System		
Case 6	Case Summary	Diabetes mellitus
Case 24	Discharge Summary	Diabetes mellitus and hypothyroidism
The Reproductive Systems		
Case 4	Ultrasound Report	Prostate ultrasound
Case 16	Operative Report	Cesarean section
Case 19	Operative Report	Modified radical mastectomy
Diagnostic Procedures		
Case 3	Radiology Report	Chest x-ray
Case 4	Ultrasound Report	Prostate ultrasound
Case 13	Operative Report	Total colonoscopy
Case 14	Operative Report	Cystoscopy

Figure 4 (*continued*)

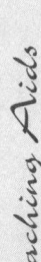

Each study is followed by five short questions that are designed to (1) encourage students to study the reports closely, (2) illustrate how diseases such as diabetes mellitus and cancer affect multiple body systems, (3) encourage students to use reference resources to locate the meanings of unfamiliar abbreviations and terms, and (4) serve as the basis of classroom discussion of the case.

Case Study Organization

Case 1, which is an excellent introduction to case studies, is unique in that it follows one patient through three types of reports for the diagnosis and treatment of appendicitis. The other studies are arranged by type of report:

- History and physical examinations
- Laboratory reports
- Case summaries
- Consultation reports
- Operative reports
- Discharge summaries

Suggestions

- **Class Discussion.** Case studies are a great way to get a class discussion going to help students better understand the relationship of the medical terms they are studying as these terms are applied to real patients.
- **Spelling Practice.** A case study can be used as a source of terms for spelling practice. As you read the case study to the students, when you come to one of the spelling words you have selected instruct students to record it on their papers.
- **Teaching Types of Reports.** These studies clearly illustrate the types of reports and the importance of each section of the report.
- **Case Study Translation.** Provide students with a copy of a case study. Have the students read the case carefully and then write a brief summary of it in "lay" terms as if they were explaining a medical condition to a patient or family member.
- **Learning More.** Assign a case study, then encourage students to do research to learn more about the diseases or conditions affecting this patient. (See Resource Files on page 20.)
- **Abbreviations.** These reports contain many abbreviations. It is important that students learn to select the correct meaning for each abbreviation based on the context of the report.
- **Complex Medical Terms.** These reports include complex terms, such as the names of syndromes or procedures, that may not have been covered in class. Finding these terms is an excellent opportunity for students to improve their skills in medical dictionary use.
- **Laboratory Tests.** These reports include many the names of laboratory tests that may be unfamiliar to the students. Finding these tests is an excellent opportunity for students to improve their skills in the use of medical resources.
- **Medications.** Many medications are mentioned in the case studies. If applicable to your course, have students use the appropriate resources to find the primary use of each medication.

COMPUTER TEACHING AIDS

Computer teaching aids are one of the most exciting new developments in teaching medical terminology as more and better programs become available. The following are some of the resources that are already on the market.

- **Delmar's Medical Terminology Challenge Software** by Pucillo. This game is fun and a great teaching tool! Students can play alone, in pairs, or in teams to try to achieve a perfect score of 2400 points. Order number 0-8273-6675-2.
- **Flash! Medical Terminology Flashcard Software.** This 500 flashcard-type question and answer program, for Windows 3.1, is organized into 16 systems and specialties. Order number 0-8273-7735-5.
- **Delmar's Anatomy and Physiology Challenge Software** by Pucillo. This game is an excellent resource for students who need additional help with the anatomy and physiology aspects of medical terminology. Order number 0-8273-7937-4.
- **Student Practice Disk** to accompany Ehrlich's *Medical Terminology for Health Professions*, 3rd ed. Each chapter unit contains four types of exercises, and a group of "Fun and Games." All provide students with instant feedback and are designed for use as additional practice or review. The questions included on the disk are *not* the same as those in the text. Fun and Games, which are actually educational, can be played by a student alone or working in pairs. The Student Practice Disk is included with the textbook.
- **Computerized Test Bank.** Many medical terminology textbooks from Delmar are accompanied by an electronic test bank. The computerized test bank to accompany *Medical Terminology for Health Professions*, 3rd edition contains over 2,000 questions drawn from the exercises in the text and from the Chapter tests in the Instructor's Guide. Order number 0-8273-7841-6.
- **Word Wizard: A Medical Terminology Software Program** by Johnson and Johnson. This program, which is divided into body systems, may provide the remedial help needed by some of your students. IBM format. Order number 0-8273-5906-3.
- **Medical Terminology CD-ROM: A Visual Guide** by Masters. Brings sight, sound, and animation to medical terminology. A particularly interesting feature is an illustrated and animated dictionary. Available in both Windows 3.1 or higher. Order number 0-8273-7734-7.

CROSSWORD PUZZLES

Medical terminology crossword puzzles and similar word search activities are another excellent way to get students to interact with the material they are learning and to have fun while practicing. Section F contains 12 crossword puzzles, and their solutions, that you are welcome to duplicate.

Suggestions

- **Student Use.** Duplicate the puzzles and let students solve them individually.
- **Class Use.** Make an overhead transparency of the puzzle and have the class work on it together as a review activity.

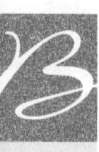

CURRENT MEDICAL INFORMATION SCRAPBOOK

A scrapbook of current medical articles is a useful classroom resource. Maintaining the scrapbook is an excellent way to encourage students to keep up-to-date on current medical articles. It is also a great way to collect material for your resource files.

Suggestions

- Select a scrapbook, with 9 x 12 pages, with page protectors that make it easy to place and remove items.
- Encourage, or assign, students to read current medical articles. This is an excellent way to make students aware of how much medical information is presented in popular newspapers and magazines.
- The student may copy the article or cut it out. Be certain that the article shows the source and date of publication.
- The article is placed in the classroom scrapbook that is available to everyone to review.
- When articles are no longer useful in the scrapbook, you may want to add them to your resource file on that topic.

Additional Suggestions

- **Reports.** Have the student present a report on the article before the article is placed in the scrapbook.
- **Duplicate.** If the article is of particular interest to the current unit being studied, make copies of it for class use with activities such as having students identify, define, and pronounce medical terms used in the article.
- **Discussion.** Periodically discuss these articles and help students learn to evaluate the accuracy of this information.

FLASH CARDS

Flash cards are a versatile teaching aid with many uses. A flash card usually has a word part on one side and the definition on the other side. For classroom use, the type on these cards should be large enough for students to see at a distance.

Suggestions

- **Do-It-Yourself.** Some teachers have students create their own flash cards because they find that this process reinforces spelling, word parts, and definitions.
- **Take-Them-Along.** Because student flash cards are small, students can select the ones applicable to their current studies and carry these cards with them. Then they can review these cards at odd times such as while waiting in line.
- **Activity Cards.** Activity cards are a variety of flash card. Both are useful in many classroom activities. (See section 6 "Activity Cards.")
- **New Varieties.** You may want to investigate the exciting new computer program called Flash! Medical Terminology Flash Card software.

FILL IN THE BLANKS

Fill in the blank activities are a good way to have students translate back and forth from medical to lay terms.

Suggestions

- **Case Studies.** Use case studies as the starting point to create a Fill-In the blank activity by either giving students the medical term and asking for the definition, or vice versa.
- **Medical Stories.** Write a brief medical story using medical or lay terms. After each term, leave a blank that the student must fill in. The story should make medical sense and may relate to typical work experiences.

Sample Story

The following is based on a story by Sandra Stevens titled "My Day at the Office." The answers are: (1) gastralgia, (2) dyspepsia, (3) gastritis, (4) gastropexy, (5) hemorrhage or hemorrhaging, (6) cyanosis, (7) dyspnea, (8) epigastric, (9) hypoglycemia, and (10) diabetic retinopathy.

MY DAY AT THE OFFICE

Welcome back to the office! Today is heavily scheduled and just as you arrive the phone rings. As you answer Mrs. D. is complaining of **pain in her stomach** (1) _____ and **indigestion** (2) _____. She thinks she may have an **inflammation of her stomach** (3) _____.

Your first scheduled patient is Mr. E. who on his last visit was postoperative from a **surgical fixation of his stomach** (4) _____. During his surgery Mr. E. had a problem with a **bursting forth of blood (excessive bleeding)** (5) _____, but that was corrected during surgery. You notice as he comes in that he has a **blueness around his skin, lips, and nailbeds** (6) _____. Your next observation is that after coming into the office he is having **difficulty breathing** (7) _____. Mr. E. quickly tells you, between breaths, that he is having some pain in the **region above his stomach** (8) _____. You promptly place this patient on a table and notify the physician of his symptoms. You are told to immediately call the squad to transfer this patient to the hospital for admission.

The next scheduled appointment is for Mr. F. who has **excessive sugar in his blood** (9) _____. He also has a **disorder of the blood vessels in the retina** (10) _____ _____ that developed as a complication of this disorder.

OVERHEAD TRANSPARENCIES

Overhead transparencies are a versatile visual aid. Section I contains 28 pieces of unlabeled art that you are welcome to duplicate to create transparencies for classroom use. To find labels, looks for similar illustrations in Ehrlich's *Medical Terminology for Health Professions*, 3rd ed.

Suggestions

- **Label size.** When creating your own transparencies with labels, be certain to use a large enough typeface (at least 12 point) so the labels can be read at a distance.

- **Add color.** Use of colored pens (specific for this purpose), to add labels, color sections, or to trace a process during class.

- **Case Studies.** can be duplicated as overhead transparencies for class discussion.

- **Testing.** Make a photocopy of the transparency art. Add appropriate lines and question numbers for the testing situation, then make a transparency of the modified art. Before use, check that the lines and numbers are clear when projected.

- **Discussion Questions.** Prepare an overhead with questions for class discussion. Use a piece of paper to cover the questions and then slide the paper to reveal the question as you are ready to discuss it.

- **Student Copies.** Some teachers provide students with printed copies of their transparencies. Students use these to take notes, color, and visualize the material. As an example, on a diagram of the heart, students actually trace the flow of blood through the heart.

PERSONAL EXPERIENCES

Contact with other people's personal experiences helps students recognize that the medical terminology they are learning is useful and essential to their success in the heathcare career of their choice.

If students are not already enrolled in a specific career track, this course can introduce them to health careers they may have not yet considered.

Guest Speakers

Having health care professionals as guest speakers is one way of helping students see this relationship. These speakers also make the class more interesting and help students better understand the topics being studied.

When arranging for a guest speaker, prepare a list of questions or topics you want the speaker to cover and give these to the speaker in advance. Also be certain that the speaker knows exactly where, when, and how long the class meets.

With the speaker's permission, have a videotape made of the presentation. This can be kept on file for future use. After the class, it is courteous to send a thank you note to the speaker.

Relating to the Real World

If you come to teaching from a health care career, you undoubtedly have extensive personal experience in the field. Sharing these experiences can be a valuable tool in illustrating the terms being discussed.

Field Trips

A field trip can help students gain valuable insights, and such an outing is often used as a reward at the end of the course. Even a picnic can be made into a fun learning experience (see the activity in Section C) "Watermelon Surgery."

PUZZLING PAIRS

Many medical terms sound alike and/or are contrasting in meaning. A list posted on the bulletin board can help students master these "puzzling pairs."

Suggestions

- **Post Them.** At the beginning of the course, post a large paper on the bulletin board titled "Puzzling pairs." Figure 5 is a sample list to help you get started.
- **Enlarge the list.** As pairs are encountered, add them to the list.
- **Use the List.** This list may be used for drills and other classroom activities.
- **Test on It.** Encourage students to study the list, and you may want to include these terms in a testing situation. Even if students can see the list on the bulletin board, they must still be able to supply the meaning of each term in the pair.

Sample Puzzling Pairs List

Abduction	⟷	Adduction
Afferent	⟷	Efferent
Anterior	⟷	Posterior
Aphasia	⟷	Asphyxia
Concussion	⟷	Contusion
Diagnosis	⟷	Prognosis
Endemic	⟷	Epidemic
Fissure	⟷	Fistula
Ileum	⟷	Ilium
Laceration	⟷	Lesion
Palpation	⟷	Palpitation
Perineum	⟷	Peritoneum
Prostate	⟷	Prostrate
Trauma	⟷	Triage
Viral	⟷	Virile

Figure 5

RESOURCE FILES

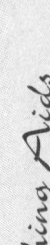

Having your personal set of resource files is an excellent tool when you need ideas and enrichment materials for class planning.

Suggestions on How to Get Started

- Create a file folder for each major topic such as the body systems and major diseases.
- File folders, with expandable sides, work best for this purpose because they keep small items from falling out.
- Arrange files in alphabetical order and allow space for adding more topics to your system.
- As you come across information on a topic, add it to the file. This might be a newspaper item, a journal article, a patient education brochure, or an idea for a class activity.
- Encourage, or assign, students to find relevant materials for addition to these files. (See "Search and Report" on page 21)

Patient Education Materials

Patient education booklets are a wonderful enrichment resource regarding specific disorders and syndromes. These booklets are usually free in limited quantities and inexpensive for larger quantities. Look for booklets published by support groups, government agencies, medical specialty organizations, and drug companies.

The **Encyclopedia of Associations**, published by Gale Research, an International Thomson Publishing Company, is an excellent source of information to locate the appropriate organizations. Most libraries include this series in their reference sections. You will want to look under the heading of "Health and Medical Organizations."

On-Line Information

If you are "on-line" with the Internet, you will find many interesting health information sources. Before adding this information to your file, evaluate the accuracy and consider carefully who or what organization provided the data.

Health Newsletters

Another excellent source of information is the better health information newsletters. Two of the most popular ones are

- *Mayo Clinic Health Letter*, Subscription Services 1-800-333-9037. In 1996, the cost was $24 per year.
- *Harvard Health Letter*, Subscription Services 1-800-829-9045. In 1996, the cost was $32 per year.

A collection of these newsletters over several years is a great resource, and the December issue usually includes an index for the year. For use in your resource files, make a photocopy of the issue, cut it apart and place the topics in the appropriate file folders.

Resources from This Kit

Many of the resources on this kit are specific for a body system. You may want to make an extra copy of each and add it to the appropriate resource file. As an example, Section H "Case Studies" has a special cross reference so you can identify cases by applicable body systems. You may want to make an extra copy of each case study and add it to the appropriate file.

SEARCH AND REPORT

Having students produce reports is a valuable teaching aid that provides them with experience in seeking out information. The resulting reports also provide enrichment materials for the entire class.

Suggestions

- Assign students to find a medical article that interests them. These articles can be from medical journals, newspapers, or magazines.

- The student should make a copy of the article and submit it with the report.

- The student is to study the article and prepare to tell the class about it.

- Make this assignment well in advance so students have time to find an article that interests them. Explain that each student must find a different article and that duplication will not be permitted.

- Have students report their topic to you as soon as it is selected. In case of duplication, the first one to report the topic gets to use the article.

Alternative Suggestions

- Assign specific articles from your "Resource File." Provide each student with a copy of an assigned topic.

- If the article is written in lay terms, have students circle these terms and be prepared to substitute the appropriate medical term.

- If the article is written in medical terms, have students circle these terms and be prepared to explain the term.

- Instead of presenting a report in class, have each student submit a written report (with a copy of the article).

STUDY SUGGESTIONS

Your students may need help getting started in learning how to study medical terminology. Figure 6 is a modified list of suggestions developed by Connie Dempsey. You might want to go over this list with your students at the beginning of the course, or you could duplicate it to be included with the course outline and syllabus.

Medical Terminology Study Suggestions

1. Study the text and complete the exercises at the end of each chapter.
2. Do not try to learn all the words in one night before the test! This will be too much to remember and you will not recall the information after the course is completed.
3. Study regularly, perhaps a half-hour to an hour per day.
4. Do not allow the amount to be learned overwhelm you! Break the chapters into smaller segments and master one or two segments per study session.
5. Make flash cards, carry them with you, and use them whenever you have a few moments to wait.
6. If you have an audiotape, listen to it often. If you do not have a tape, consider creating your own.
7. Say the words and definitions aloud. Repeat this process many times.
8. Write the words and their definitions. Repeat this process many times.
9. In addition to your assignments, do medical terminology puzzles or play related computer games. The more you use the words, the easier it becomes.
10. Form a study group with other medical terminology students and quiz each other.

Figure 6

TEAM AND CLASS ACTIVITIES

At times team activities invigorate a class. Other times an activity involving the entire class is your best choice. Section C contains may activities. Below is a listing that will help you select activities best suited for each type of situation.

Team Activities	Class Activities
Alphabet Soup	Aerobic Action
Bowl Games	Bingo
Create-a-Word	Body Planes and Directions
Definition Bee	Concentration
Human Word Building	Create-a-Word
Jeopardy!®	Hangman
Labeling Body Parts	Random Access
Medical Term Dissection	Spelling Bee
Medical Terminology Challenge	Term or Definition?
Speed Writing	The Living Heart
Spelling Bee	Twenty Questions
Terminology Battle	Understanding Afferent and Efferent Neurons
Watermelon Surgery	Watermelon Surgery

VIDEOTAPES

Videotapes are a wonderful way to help students better visualize the body system or other topics under discussion.

Suggestions

- One such series is *The Human Machine* from National Geographic.
- Another source of useful videotapes is patient education materials that explain a condition or procedure in simple terms for a layperson. Many such tapes are produced by medical specialty groups and by companies specializing in patient education materials.
- A teaching hospital may be a source of videotapes showing specific procedures, such as a laparoscopic cholecystectomy, in detail. Educational TV channels may also air tapes of this type.
- Many hospitals also have a patient education library that includes videos to teach patients with specific conditions how to care for themselves (e.g., a video on ostomy care).
- Although you may not have class time to show these videos, you can make them available as enrichment materials to students who are interested. Another alternative is to assign students to watch different tapes (in the library), and then to report to the class.

VISUAL AIDS

Many visual aids are available to help your students grasp complex concepts as they are learning medical terminology.

Suggestions

- **Wall Charts.** The classic wall chart really is effective—if the print and pictures are large enough for students to see.
- **Bulletin Board.** As you start the study of a new body system, post appropriate illustrations and articles on the bulletin board. (See Resource Files on page 20.)
- **Anatomic Models.** Anatomic models with removable body parts can also be effective visual aids. If you do not have access to models from traditional sources, look for kits, such as the visible woman, in a hobby shop or toy store.
- **Additional Aids.** Overhead transparencies, slides, videotapes, and some computer animation programs are also excellent visual aids.

WRITE-A-STORY

This class assignment is an interesting way to have students work with the terms they are learning.

Suggestions

- Students are to write a very short story using 5 to 10 terms from the chapter being studied. You may provide a list of assigned words or you may allow students to select the terms.
- The story need not be true, and students are welcome to make it funny; however, the use of the terms must be medically correct.
- If there is time, students can share their stories with the class.

SECTION C

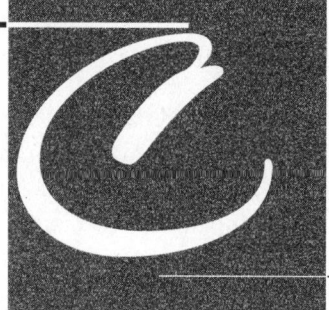

Classroom Activities

Overview of Classroom Activities

1. **Aerobic Action**—This class activity helps students learn about muscle movements by actually performing them.

2. **Alphabet Soup**—This team activity allows students to have fun while they learn commonly used medical abbreviations.

3. **Bingo**—This is a popular class activity. Ready to photocopy and use Word Part Bingo can be found in Section D.

4. **Body Planes And Directions**—This class activity aids students in learning the names of body planes and directions through related movements.

5. **Bowl Games**—This class activity is similar to TV college bowls. This competition can be carried on throughout an entire course.

6. **Concentration**—This class activity is a modification of the classic card game and uses medical terminology flashcards.

7. **Create-A-Word**—This activity allows students to have fun creating nonsense words using actual medical word parts. Version #1 is a team activity. Version #2 is small group activity.

8. **Definition Bee**—This team activity is an alternative way for students to practice defining medical terms.

9. **Hangman**—This version of the classic hangman game is fun, requires no advance preparation, and can be played either as a class or small group activity.

10. **Human Word Building**—This team activity combines the fun of moving around with the challenge of building actual medical terms.

11. **Jeopardy!®**—This is a medical terminology version of Jeopardy!® the television quiz show. Ready to photocopy and play Word Part Jeopardy! and Body System Jeopardy! can be found in Section E.

12. **Labeling Body Parts**—This team activity encourages students to have fun while practicing associating combining forms with actual body parts. Version #1 has students draw a body on the board. Inversion #2 students work with an anatomic model.

13. **Medical Term Dissection**—This team activity gives students practice in analyzing complex medical terms by dissecting the terms into word parts.
14. **Medical Terminology Challenge**—This team activity challenges students to either correctly spell, define, or identify a medical term presented by the other team.
15. **Random Access**—This class activity provides students with opportunities to spell and define terms.
16. **Scrabble®**—This medical terminology version of Scrabble® can be played as a small group activity.
17. **Speed Writing**—This team activity is an excellent review that also allows the instructor to determine how well students are prepared for an examination.
18. **Spelling Bee**—This activity is a great way to make spelling practice more fun. Version #1 is a class activity. Versions #2 and #3 are played with teams.
19. **Terminology Battle**—This team activity helps students have fun while they review medical term definitions, pronunciations, and spelling.
20. **Term Or Definition?**—This class activity challenges students to either correctly spell, define, or identify a medical term presented by a classmate.
21. **Terminology Pursuit**—This small group activity is a medical version of the board game Trivial Pursuit®.
22. **The Living Heart**—In this class activity students portray the flow of blood through the heart. Taking part in the experience clarifies this difficult concept and helps students remember it.
23. **Twenty Questions**—This variation on a familiar game is a good review activity for the entire class.
24. **Understanding Afferent And Efferent Neurons**—This class activity helps students visualize and experience the roles of afferent and efferent neurons.
25. **Watermelon Surgery**—This team activity is fun at a class outing, such as a picnic or party.

AEROBIC ACTION

Purpose: This class activity helps students learn about muscle movements by actually performing them. Version #1 has the cadence of a drill team. Version #2 is organized like an aerobic workout and you may want to find music to accompany it.

Advance Preparation

- Determine what sort of action can be used to represent each type of muscle movement. (Arms-only actions are better in a limited space.)
- List the muscle movements on the board: abduction and adduction; flexion and extension; elevation and depression; rotation and circumduction; supination and pronation.

The Activity, Version #1

- Have students stand far enough apart to allow for arm movements.
- Review the terms and the movement that represents each one.
- Randomly call the types of motions. As a term is called, students make the appropriate movement.

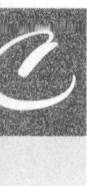

- Each time you go through the list pick up the pace.
- *Optional:* Make the final rounds competitive; a student who makes the wrong movement must sit down and is out of the game.

The Activity, Version #2

- Have students stand far enough apart to allow for arm movements.
- Review the terms and the movement that represents each one.
- Give the terms like instructions for an aerobic workout. Start with clues such as "Elevate, bring them up. Flexion, bend them in."
- As you progress through the workout, drop the clues about the movements, and speed up the pace.

ALPHABET SOUP

Purpose: This team activity allows students to have fun while they learn commonly used medical abbreviations.

Advance Preparation

- Prepare a list of abbreviations and their meanings.
- Have reference books available to look up contested answers.

The Activity, Version #1

- Divide the class into two teams. Have them stand in two lines. A coin toss determines which team goes first.
- The leader (teacher) writes an abbreviation on the board.
- The player at the head of the line must state the meaning of the abbreviation within 20 seconds. The team may confer and use reference books.
- If the answer is correct, the player moves to the end of the line and it is the other team's turn.
- If the answer is incorrect, that player is out of the game and the other team is given a chance at the abbreviation.
- The team with the most players left at the end of a fixed number of rounds wins.

The Activity, Version #2

- Divide the class into two teams. Have them stand in two lines. A coin toss determines which team goes first.
- The leader (teacher) writes an abbreviation on the board.
- The player at the head of the line must state the meaning of the abbreviation within 10 seconds.
- If the answer is correct, the player moves to the end of the line and it is the other team's turn.

- If the answer is incorrect, that player is out of the game and the other team is given a chance at the abbreviation.
- The winners are the team with the most players left at the end of a fixed number of rounds.

BINGO

Purpose: This class activity is fun and it helps students practice medical word parts. A ready to photocopy and play version of Word Part Bingo is located in Section D.

BODY PLANES AND DIRECTIONS

Purpose: This class activity helps students learn the names of body planes and directions through related movements. Version #2 is a variation of "Simon Says." The goal in both versions is to keep all of the students involved as long as possible.

Advance Preparation

- Determine what action can be used to represent each term. (See list of suggested movements.)
- List on the board the body planes to be demonstrated: sagittal, coronal (frontal), and horizontal (transverse).
- List on the board the body directions to be demonstrated: ventral and dorsal, anterior and posterior, superior and inferior, cephalic and caudal, distal and medial.

Suggested Movements

- **Sagittal plane**—Up and down hand movement, as if cutting, with fingers pointing at the midline or long axis of the body.
- **Coronal plane**—Up and down hand movement, as if cutting, with fingers pointing at the side of the body.
- **Horizontal plane**—Side to side hand movement, as if cutting, at the waist.
- **Ventral** and **anterior**—Pat the front of the body.
- **Dorsal** and **posterior**—Pat the back of the body.
- **Superior** and **cephalic**—Raise the arm and point upward.
- **Inferior** and **caudal**—Lower the arm and point downward.
- **Proximal**—Touch the humerus (upper arm) near the shoulder.
- **Distal**—Touch the humerus (upper arm) near the elbow.
- **Medial**—Point toward the midline (middle of the body).
- **Lateral**—Point toward the side away from the midline (middle of the body).

The Activity, Version #1

- Have students stand far enough apart to allow for arm movements.
- Review the terms and the movement that represents each one.

- Call the terms in random order. As each term is called, students make the appropriate movement.
- Each time you go through the list pick up the pace.
- *Optional:* Make the final rounds competitive, a student who makes the wrong movement must sit down and is out of the game.

The Activity, Version #2

- Have students stand far enough apart to allow for arm movements.
- Review the terms and the movement that represents each one.
- Players are to respond only to a command beginning with "Simon Says." Anyone giving a wrong response or responding to a command that does not begin with "Simon Says" is eliminated from the game.
- With each round, increase the pace of the activity.

BOWL GAMES

Purpose: This team activity, which is based on TV college bowl games, involves the entire class in a competition that can be carried on throughout an entire course.

At the beginning of the term divide the class into three teams. Each team may want to adopt a name and appoint a captain or spokesperson. When the game is played, two teams compete and the third team acts as the scorekeepers and audience. The audience is expected to fully participate by applauding and trying to guess the answers.

Advance Preparation

- **Questions.** Prepare 50 to 60 questions and answers. An alternative is to select appropriate activity cards and flashcards and have the game host phrase the term as a question.
- **Competitors.** Determine which two teams are to compete and which is to be the audience for this round.
- **Scorekeepers** and audience. From the third team, appoint a scorekeeper for each of the competing teams. Scores are recorded on the board where everyone can see them. The remaining members of that team serve as the audience.
- **Game Host.** The teacher usually acts as the game host.

The Activity, Version #1

- The game host reads the first question.
- Participants respond as quickly as possible by raising their hands. In case of conflict, the game host determines which hand went up first.
- Team members may not confer. If the team member responding first gets the correct answer, that team is awarded +5 points and the game progresses to the next definition.
- If the team member responding first does not get the correct answer, that team is awarded -5 points and the other team is given an opportunity to give the right answer.

- If neither team gets it right, the game host gives the correct answer and goes on to the next question.
- The game is played for the predetermined length of time. A winner for the day is announced and team scores are recorded toward the championship.

The Activity, Version #2

- A coin toss determines which team gets the first question. Team members may confer on the answer; however, reference materials may not be used.
- The team leader gives the response. If the answer is right, the team is awarded +5 points.
- If the answer is not correct, the team is awarded -5 points and the question goes to the other team.
- If neither team gets it right, the game host gives the correct answer and goes on to the next question.
- The game is over when time is up or the moderator runs out of questions. If the teams are tied, a really difficult term is used as the tiebreaker.

CONCENTRATION

Purpose: This class activity is a modification of the classic card game and uses medical terminology flash cards.

Advance Preparation

- A conference table is necessary so the cards can be spread out.
- Two matching "sets" of flashcards are needed for this activity. These flashcards have a word part on one side and the definition on the other.
- One set of flashcards is placed in a pile in the middle of the table with the definition up and the word part down.
- The second set of flashcards is spread around on the table with the definition side up.

The Activity

- Students stand around the table.
- The caller pulls a card from the bottom of the pile (so the other players will not see either side before the play begins). The caller reveals the word part shown on the card.
- The first student who finds the correct definition for the word part slaps that card and removes it from the table.
- This student gets to reveal the next card.
- The student with the most cards wins.

CREATE-A-WORD

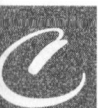

Purpose: This activity allows students to have fun creating nonsense words using actual medical word parts. Version #1 is a team activity. Version #2 is small group activity.

Advance Preparation

- Have available reference books where students can find medical word parts.
- An alternative is to provide flashcards or a list of assigned word parts that may be used.
- For version #1 divide the class into teams of about 5 members each.
- Version #2 requires the preparation of instructions for each group.

Guidelines

1. These should *not* be real medical terms; however, they must be made of medical word parts.
2. The terms may be humorous, lengthy, and deliberately difficult.
3. The terms must follow spelling rules and have a logical definition.
4. The list of terms must be completed within the time allotted (10 minutes is recommended).

The Activity, Version #1

- Each team is to work with medical word parts to "create" five words according to the guidelines shown above. (Allow about 5 to 10 minutes for this.)
- The teams take turns writing a newly created word on the board. Other teams compete to guess the definition first. Points are awarded for each correct answer.
- After all terms have been presented, the entire class votes for "the best" (most creative) term devised by a team. Extra points are awarded for this and the team with the most points wins.

The Activity, Version #2

- Students work in groups of two to three.
- Give each group a set of instructions such as "Make any word that means to surgically repair."
- The groups have 3 minutes to generate a list of applicable terms. These can be actual terms or nonsense words; however, no books or references are allowed.
- At the end of the time, groups share their lists.

DEFINITION BEE

Purpose: This team activity is an alternative way for students to practice defining medical terms.

Advance Preparation

- Create a list of words to be defined (preferably at least two terms per student)
- Divide the class into two teams.
- The instructor acts as the caller.

The Activity, Version #1

- A coin toss determines which team goes first.
- The caller gives team A a term they must define within 20 seconds. (Teams are allowed to confer on the answer.)
- If the team answers correctly and within the time, team A is awarded 5 points.
- If the team is unable to answer correctly, the term goes to team B.
- Play continues as the caller gives team B a term they must define within 20 seconds.
- The team with the most points wins.

The Activity, Version #2

- Have the teams stand in lines.
- A coin toss determines which team goes first.
- The caller gives the first member of team A a term to be defined within 15 seconds. (Teams are *not* allowed to confer on the answer)
- If the answer is correct and within the time, team A is awarded 5 points and the player goes to the back of the line.
- If the answer is not correct, that player is out of the game and the term goes to team B.
- Play continues as the caller gives the first member of team B a term to be defined within 15 seconds.
- The team with the most remaining players wins.

HANGMAN

Purpose: This version of the classic hangman game is quick and fun. Version #1 is played with the entire class using the chalkboard. Version #2 is a "seat activity" for groups of two or three students.

Advance Preparation

- **Establish the rules.** The most common version of this game has a body drawn in six steps (head, body, arm, arm, leg, leg).
- When working with longer words, more opportunities can be provided by having the hangman draw hands and feet—even fingers and toes.
- You may want to specify the topic and the maximum or minimum word length.

The Activity, Version #1

- Explain the rules and the object of the game, which is to guess the word before the hanging is complete.
- Designate a hangman who thinks of an appropriate term. You can fill this role or have students take turns doing it.
- On the chalk board, the hangman draws the scaffold and noose and then writes a series of dashes to indicate the number of letters in the word. For example, the lines for **cardiorrhexis** would look like this __ __ __ __ __ __ __ __ __ __ __ __ .
- The other players guess the letters of the word, calling out one letter at a time.
- If the letter occurs in the word, the hangman writes the letter above the appropriate dash wherever that letter occurs.
- If the letter does not occur in the word, the incorrect letter is recorded underneath the dashes. This way the players can see which letters have been tried.
- For each wrong guess, the hangman draws a part of the hangman picture.
- The player who guesses the word before the hangman picture is complete is declared the winner **if** he or she can correctly pronounce and define the term. The winner becomes the hangman for the next round.
- If the other players do not guess the word before the hangman picture is completed, the hangman is declared the winner **if** he or she can correctly spell, pronounce, and define the term.
- If he or she cannot do this, another player is automatically the hangman for the next round.

The Activity, Version #2

- A small group of students quietly carry out the hangman activities using pencil and paper.
- Each game is played on a separate paper showing the name of the hangman, the term, and the name of the winner. These papers are given to the teacher at the end of the activity.

HUMAN WORD BUILDING

Purpose: This team activity combines the fun of moving around with the challenge of building actual medical terms.

Advance Preparation

- Select the flashcards. Each group should receive *at least* two prefixes, four combining forms, and six suffixes.
- Divide the class into teams of up to six members.

The Activity

- Give each team their flashcards.

- Allow teams 5 minutes to find words that can be created from these word parts. Dictionaries and reference materials are encouraged. As terms are discovered, they should be recorded on paper by the team.
- Teams take turns presenting words by having students hold cards and line up to create a term. The team must also be able to define the term.
- After a word has been presented and defined correctly, it is recorded on the board under the team's name. (It must be spelled correctly to count.)
- Teams take turns until all terms have been given.
- The team with the most correct terms wins.

JEOPARDY!®

Purpose: This popular team activity is a medical terminology version of Jeopardy!® the television quiz show. Ready to photocopy and play Word Part Jeopardy! and Body System Jeopardy! can be found in Section E.

LABELING BODY PARTS

Purpose: This team activity encourages students to have fun while practicing associating combining forms with actual body parts. Version #1 has students draw a body on the board. In version #2 students work with an anatomic model.

Advance Preparation

- Prepare a list of combining forms (see suggested list below).
- Divide the class into two teams.
- Version #2 requires an anatomic model, Post-It™ notes in two colors, and two lists of combining forms.

Suggested Word Part List: *ABDOMIN/O, ARTHR/O, CARDI/O, COL/O, COST/O, CRANI/O, CUTANE/O, ENTER/O, ESOPHAG/O, GASTR/O, HEPAT/O, MY/O, OCUL/O, OR/O, OT/O, PNEUM/O, REN/O, RHIN/O, SPLEN/O THORAC/O, TRACHE/O,* and *THYROID/O.*

The Activity, Version #1

- Give each team a copy of the body part combining form list.
- Have one member of each team draw a large outline of the upper body on the board.
- Teams are allowed 2 minutes to look up the meaning of the combining forms.
- At the signal to start, each team as quickly as possible draws an "X" to represent the body part and labels it with the appropriate combining form.
- The first team finished gets to present their "body" by identifying each combining form and what it represents.
- The second team then gets to present their "body" by identifying each combining form and what it represents.

- If the first team finished gives accurate answers, it is the winner.
- If the first team finished does not give accurate answers and the other team does, they are the winners.
- If neither team get all answers correct, the team with the most accurate responses wins.

The Activity, Version #2

- Provide different colored Post-It™ notes for each team. Also give each team a different list of combining forms.
- Allow teams 2 minutes to look up the meaning of the combining forms and to write one combining form on each Post-It™ note to create a body part label.
- A coin toss determines which team goes first.
- Team A quickly places a label on the appropriate body part. Then, team B quickly places a label on the appropriate body part.
- Teams take turns until all body parts are labeled.
- Team A is given an opportunity to identify a body part labeled by team B by stating and spelling the combining form. If the answer is correct, they get to remove the label.
- Team B is given an opportunity to identify a body part labeled by team A by stating and spelling the combining form. If the answer is correct, they get to remove the label.
- At the end of play, the team with the most labels wins.

MEDICAL TERM DISSECTION

Purpose: This team activity gives students practice in analyzing complex medical terms by dissecting the terms into word parts.

Advance Preparation

- Create cards of medical terms made up of combinations of word parts. You will need one per student.
- Divide the class into teams of four to five students.
- Give each team member at least one word card.

The Activity

- Each team appoints one team member as the clue giver. (This role moves around the team circle.)
- The clue giver gives clues based on the word parts in the term. The rest of the team tries to guess the word within 10 seconds. They must also be able to pronounce, spell, and define the term.
- If their answer is correct, the next team member becomes the clue giver and the process is repeated.
- If the team cannot guess a term correctly, the card is removed from the circle.

- At the end of the round, unanswered cards are returned.
- In a bonus round, these cards are distributed to the other teams. If they give the correct answer, they keep the card.
- The team with the most cards wins.

MEDICAL TERMINOLOGY CHALLENGE

Purpose: This team activity challenges students to either correctly spell, define, or identify a medical term presented by the other team. ("Term or Definition?" on page 39 is the class version of this activity.)

Advance Preparation

- Activity cards, flashcards, or a combination of both may be used. Select at least one card for each team member.
- Divide the class into two teams. These teams are described here as A and B; however, students may enjoy adopting a team name.

The Activity, Version #1

- A coin toss determines which team goes first.
- Team A selects the card to be used first and decides whether the respondent must correctly spell the term, define the term, or give the term in response to the definition. A student from team A presents this challenge to a student from team B.
- Team B is allowed 15 seconds to consult on the answer. The student who was challenged presents the answer. If the answer is correct, 10 points are awarded to the team.
- If the answer is not correct, the student who was challenged sits down and is out of the game.
- Play continues, rotating teams so each student has an opportunity to ask a question and an opportunity to answer a question.
- At the end of play, the team with the most points wins.

The Activity, Version #2

- A coin toss determines which team goes first.
- Team A selects the card to be used first and decides whether the respondent must correctly spell the term, define the term, or give the term in response to the definition. A student from team A presents this challenge to a student from team B.
- The student on team B is allotted 15 seconds to answer. Team members may not confer on the answer. If the answer is correct, 10 points are awarded to the team.
- If the answer is not correct, 5 points are subtracted from the team score.
- Play continues rotating teams so that each student has an opportunity to ask a question and an opportunity to answer a question.
- At the end of play, the team with the most points wins.

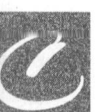

RANDOM ACCESS

Purpose: This class activity provides students with opportunities to spell and define terms. Version #2 has the advantage of added suspense because students do not know where the beanbag will be tossed next.

Advance Preparation

- Prepare one word slip for each class member. Each slip may be *either* a term or a definition.
- Version #1, place prepared slips in a brown bag.
- Version #2 requires a beanbag or similar soft object to toss from one player to another.

The Activity, Version #1

- Taking turns, each student pulls out a word slip and responds within 15 seconds.
- If the slip contains a term, the student must define it. If the slip contains a definition, the student must identify and spell the term.
- If the student does not answer correctly, the teacher gives the correct answer and moves on to the next student.

The Activity, Version #2

- The players are seated in a circle and each is given a word slip.
- The first player, who is holding the beanbag, tosses the beanbag to another player. The first player then reads the term or definition from his or her word slip.
- The player receiving the beanbag must respond within 15 seconds. If the slip contains a term, the student must define it. If the slip contains a definition, the student must identify and spell the term.
- After the question has been answered, that player gets to toss the beanbag and asks the question from his or her word slip. After the question has been answered, the player who tossed the beanbag is out of the game. (This way each student receives the beanbag only once.)

SCRABBLE®

Purpose: A medical terminology version of Scrabble® can be played as a small group activity.

Advance Preparation

- A Scrabble® set (Milton Bradley Company, a subsidiary of Hasbro, Inc., Springfield, MA 01101).
- Prepare the modified rules and keep a copy of them with the game set.

The Modified Rules

- Only medical terms are allowed.
- Each player draws 10 tiles.
- Players must define words as they play them. If the definition is not correct, no score is given for the word.
- A medical dictionary and other references may be used but the move must be completed within 1 minute.
- Disputed terms must be found in an accepted reference source.

The Activity

- Up to four players are allowed in the game.
- Play proceeds according to the modified rules.

SPEED WRITING

Purpose: This team activity is an excellent review that also allows the instructor to determine how well students are prepared for an examination.

Advance Preparations

- Determine the words to be used.
- Divide the class into two teams and have each team stand in line.

The Activity

- Each team positions a player at the board.
- The teacher dictates a medical term.
- The player who is first to spell the word correctly on the board wins a point for his or her team. Both players go to the back of their team line and the next player comes to the board.
- If neither player spells the term correctly, no points are awarded and the next pair of players tries again.
- This round continues until all team members have participated once.
- In the next round the teacher gives the definition only.
- The players must supply and spell the term. For the answer to be correct, the player must also pronounce the term correctly.
- Play continues until all team members have participated again.
- The team with the most points wins.

SPELLING BEE

Purpose: This activity is a great way to make spelling practice more fun. Version #1 is a class activity. Versions #2 and #3 are played with teams.

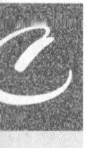

Advance Preparation

- **Prepare a word list.** The list should include the definition and correct pronunciation for each word. Usually the list begins with easier terms and progresses to more difficult ones. There should be enough terms to go around the group more than once.
- **The caller.** Appoint a caller to give the words. This may be a student or the teacher. It is important that the caller be able to pronounce the terms correctly.
- Version #3 requires a pair of dice that are used to determine point value.

The Activity, Version #1

- All players are standing at the beginning of this game.
- The caller gives the player a word. The player must repeat the word, define it, and then spell the term.
- If the answer is correct, the player remains standing and goes to the end of the line.
- If the answer is not correct, the player is out and must sit down.
- The caller goes on to the next player. The missed term may be reused until someone gets it right.
- The last player standing is the winner.

The Activity, Version #2

- Divide the class into two teams with each team standing in a line.
- A coin toss determines which team goes first.
- The caller gives the first player from team A a word. The player must repeat the word, define it, and then spell the term.
- If the term is given, the student must pronounce it and give the definition.
- If the answer is correct, +5 points are awarded, the player adds this to the team score, then goes to the end of the team line.
- If the answer is not correct, -5 points are awarded, the player subtracts this from the team score, then goes to the end of the team line.
- The caller goes on to the next player. The missed term may be reused until someone gets it right.
- The winner is the team with the highest score at the end of play.

The Activity, Version #3

- This is played like version #2 except for the method of scoring.
- The student who is to spell the term, rolls dice for point value.
- If the student spells the word correctly, the team gets the number of points as determined by the roll of the dice.
- If the student does not spell the word correctly, the other team gets to try spelling the term for the points first rolled.
- The winner is the team with the highest score at the end of play.

TERMINOLOGY BATTLE

Purpose: This team activity helps students have fun while they review medical term definition, pronunciation, and spelling. In version #1 the challenge is to supply and spell a term based on the definition. In version #2 the challenge is to define and spell a term.

Advance Preparation

- Divide the class into two teams.
- Provide each team with the current study list of medical terms.
- Prepare a list of terms for use by each team.
- An alternative is to allow each team to generate its own list based on the current lesson.

The Activity, Version #1

- A coin toss determines which team goes first.
- Team A selects a word from their list and gives the *definition* to team B. Each term may only be used once in the game.
- Team B responds by giving the term and spelling it correctly within 15 seconds. (This may be an individual or a team effort.)
- If the answer is correct, team B is awarded +5 points and they present a definition to team A.
- If the answer is not correct, team A gives the correct answer and presents another definition to team B.
- The team with the most points wins.

The Activity, Version #2

- A coin toss determines which team goes first.
- Team A pronounces a term. (Students take turn pronouncing.) If the pronunciation is correct, team A is awarded one point.
- Team B defines the term and spells it correctly within 15 seconds. (This may be an individual or a team effort.)
- If the answer is correct, team B is awarded +5 points and they present a term to team A.
- If the answer is not correct, team A gives the correct answer and presents another term to team B.
- The team with the most points wins.

TERM OR DEFINITION?

Purpose: This class activity challenges students to either correctly spell, define, or identify a medical term presented by a classmate. (Medical Terminology Challenge is a team version of this activity.)

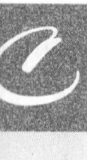

Advance Preparation

- Activity cards, flashcards, or a combination of both may be used. Select at least one card for each student and place the cards in a container such as a bowl, hat, or bag.

The Activity, Version #1

- Randomly select a student to start the game.
- The student picks a card, shows one side to the class, and selects someone to answer the question.
- If the word part or term is shown, the answer must be the definition. If the definition is shown, the answer must be the word part or term.
- If the answer is correct, that student selects and presents the next card.
- If the answer is not correct, another student is selected to try. The student giving the correct answer selects and presents the next card.
- No student is called on to answer more than once until everyone has had a chance to participate.

The Activity, Version #2

- Randomly select a student to start the game.
- That student picks a card, selects someone to answer, and then asks "Term or Definition?"
- If the respondent selects **term**, that side of the card is shown and the answer is the definition. If the respondent selects **definition**, that side of the card is shown and the answer is the term.
- If the answer is correct, that student selects and presents the next card.
- If the answer is not correct, another student is selected to try. The student giving the correct answer selects and presents the next card.
- No student is called on to answer more than once until everyone has had a chance to participate.

TERMINOLOGY PURSUIT

Purpose: This small group activity is a medical version of the board game Trivial Pursuit® in which medical terminology flashcards are substituted for the cards that come with the game.

Advance Preparation

- Obtain the game set Trivial Pursuit® (Parker Brothers, Division of Tonka Corp., Beverly, MA 01915).
- Organize a set of flashcards into categories (prefixes, combining forms, and suffixes).

Modified Rules

- Follow the game rules for movement around the board.
- A player landing on a *pink* or *brown* space draws a prefixes card.
- A player landing on a *blue* or *yellow* space draws a combining form card.
- A player landing on an *orange* or *green* space draws a suffix card.
- The player must correctly define the word part. If the answer is correct, that player moves again. If the answer is not correct, it is the next player's turn.

The Activity

- There may be up to four players.
- Set up the board and follow the modified rules for the game.

THE LIVING HEART

Purpose: In this class activity students portray the flow of blood through the heart. Seeing this flow and actively taking part in the experience clarifies this difficult concept and helps students remember it.

Advance Preparation

- List these terms on the board: superior and inferior venae cavae, right atrium, tricuspid valve, right ventricle, pulmonary semilunar valve, pulmonary artery, pulmonary veins, left ventricle, mitral valve, left atrium, aortic semilunar valve, aorta.
- Provide materials for labels or signs. A marker used to write big letters on masking tape can be used for labels.
- Have two students stand and face each other to form each of the four chambers of the heart. Name and label the chambers.
- Assign a student to be the lungs and stand slightly away from the heart. (This student can be labeled or provided with a sign to hold.)
- Assign a student to be the "blood" and stand ready to flow through the heart.
- The remaining students must answer questions to permit the blood to flow through the heart.

The Activity

- Have the chambers position themselves to form a heart and name the points at which their hands join. (Students can be provided with signs to hold.)
- The blood positions itself ready to begin its journey through the heart.
- **Question:** Blood, where are you and where do you want to go?
- **Answer:** I am in the superior and inferior venae cavae. I want to go into the right atrium.
- **Movement:** The venae cavae hands open and blood progresses into the right atrium.

- **Question:** Blood, what stands in your way and where do you want to go?
- **Answer:** The tricuspid valve is in my way, and I want to go into the right ventricle.
- **Movement:** The tricuspid valve hands open and the blood progresses into the right ventricle.
- **Question:** Blood, what stands in your way and where do you want to go?
- **Answer:** The pulmonary semilunar valve is in my way, and I want to go into the pulmonary artery.
- **Movement:** The pulmonary semilunar valve hands open and the blood progresses into the pulmonary artery and on to the lungs.
- **Question:** Blood, where are you and what are you doing?
- **Answer:** I am in the lungs giving off waste products and receiving oxygen.
- **Movement:** Blood moves back to the heart.
- **Question:** Blood, where are you and where do you want to go?
- **Answer:** I am in the pulmonary veins and I want to go into the left atrium.
- **Movement:** The pulmonary vein hands open and the blood moves into the left atrium.
- **Question:** Blood, what stands in your way and where do you want to go?
- **Answer:** The mitral valve stands in my way and I want to go to the left ventricle.
- **Movement:** The mitral hands open and the blood progresses into the left ventricle.
- **Question:** Blood, what stands in your way and where do you want to go?
- **Answer:** The aortic semilunar valve stands in my way. I want to go into the aorta and then to all parts of the body (except the lungs).
- **Movement:** The aortic semilunar valve hands open and the blood leaves the heart.
- The activity can be continued by having the blood return to the heart.

TWENTY QUESTIONS

Purpose: This variation on a familiar game is a good review activity for the entire class.

Advance Preparation

- Establish the word selection parameters such as word parts or a particular body system.
- If the topic is **word parts**, the participants are to guess whether it is a *prefix*, *combining form*, or *suffix*.
- If the topic is a **body system**, the players are to guess whether it relates to *anatomy, pathology, or procedures*.
- Appoint a scorekeeper to keep track of the number of questions asked.

The Activity

- The "leader" thinks of a medical term within the given parameters. The leader must be able to pronounce, spell, and define the selected term.

- The players must guess the word by asking questions that can be answered **yes** or **no**. The goal is to guess the term in the fewest possible questions.
- To win, the person guessing the correct term must also be able to pronounce, spell, and define it.
- This person becomes the leader for the next round.
- Points are awarded for each term correctly identified by each player.
- If the term is not guessed within 20 questions, the leader must give the term, and then spell and define it.

UNDERSTANDING AFFERENT AND EFFERENT NEURONS

Purpose: This class activity helps students visualize and experience the roles of afferent and efferent neurons. Version #1 positions the students as afferent and efferent neurons. Version #2, a variation of "whispering down the lane," demonstrates how messages travel along these pathways.

Advance Preparation

- Write these key terms on the board: neuron cell body, axon, dendrite, synapse, afferent neuron, and efferent neuron.
- Appoint one student to act as the brain. (You may want to provide a large sign or label for the brain.)
- Appoint one student to act as a muscle. (You may want to provide a large sign or label for the muscle.)

The Activity, Version #1

- As you give students instructions to position themselves, identify each role with a term on the board.
- Have students stand in a line facing forward (allow space for students to extend their arms to the side). Each student's body represents the **neuron cell body**.
- Have students extend and separate the fingers of the right hand using the index finger as a pointer. The right hand represents the **axon**.
- Have students make the left hand into a fist. The uncovered left hand is the **dendrite**.
- Have students extend both arms straight out from the body toward the side. They should be standing close enough together to almost, but not quite, touch. This space is the **synapse**.
- Have the **brain** stand at one end of the line with the last student's axon pointed toward it.
- Have the **muscle** stand at other end of the line with the last student's dendrite pointed toward it.
- Ask the students if they represent an afferent or efferent nerve. The correct response is "*afferent*."
- Have all the neurons do an about face. (The brain and muscle do not move.) Now the dendrites are pointed toward the brain.
- Ask the students if they represent an afferent or efferent nerve. The correct response is "*efferent*."

The Activity, Version #2

- With the students positioned as efferent neurons, have the muscle send a message to the brain. This is done by whispering from one efferent neuron to the next. The message might be, "*Trouble here, I need to move.*"
- After the brain receives the message, reverse positions so students are now afferent neurons, then have the brain reply. This is done by whispering from one afferent neuron to the next. The message might be, "*OK, contract and get going.*"

WATERMELON SURGERY

Purpose: This team activity is fun at a class outing, such as a picnic or party.

Advance Preparation

- Divide the class into teams. The number of teams depends on the class size. Each team should be about four to six students.
- Provide each team with an instruction sheet.
- Provide each team with a watermelon, marker, knife, long straw, and short straw.

The Activity

- Review the instruction sheet and define each of the procedures to be performed.
- Use the marker to draw an outline on the outside of the watermelon to accommodate these procedures.
- Perform the procedures as outlined on the instruction sheet.
- When teams are finished, their efforts are compared and a winner is selected. If challenged, the winning team must be able to define the procedures they have performed.
- All teams get to enjoy eating their watermelons.

WATERMELON SURGERY INSTRUCTIONS

PLEASE BE VERY CAREFUL WITH THE KNIVES!

Surgery To be Performed:

- **Abdominocentesis**—Cut a small hole and place a **long straw** in the hole.
- **Gastrotomy**—Cut an "X" to mark the spot.
- **Lumpectomy**—Cut out a square and **remove the piece**.
- **Rhinoplasty**—Cut out a square and then **replace** it in the hole.
- **Tracheostomy**—Cut a small hole and place a **short straw** in the hole.

SECTION D

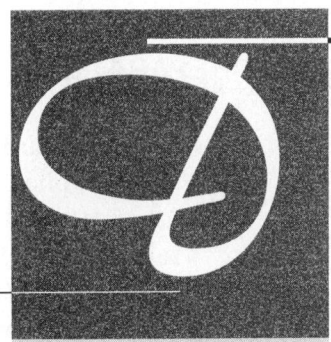

Medical Word Part Bingo

Purpose: This very popular class activity is fun and it helps students practice medical word parts. Because a player must be able to define the word parts before being declared a winner, one option is to give students copies of the word list in advance. By practicing for the game they will have mastered 50 word parts!

Because of the random nature of play, each game is different and the same supplies can be used to play at almost anytime throughout the course. However, you may want to create more versions. At the end of this game there is a blank callers list form and a blank bingo card that can be photocopied and used for this purpose.

ADVANCE PREPARATION

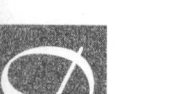

- **Bingo cards.** Included here are 10 "Medical Word Part Bingo" cards ready to be photocopied for use. Make enough copies so you have at least one card per student.
- **Markers.** With photocopied cards, markers are not required. Just have students pencil an "X" through the word part that was called. The same card can be reused by having the word part circled for the second game. If you want to use markers consider small squares of colored paper, bingo chips from commercially available games, buttons, or even M & M candies that the students get to eat at the end of class!
- **Caller's list.** The caller's list included here contains 50 commonly used medical word parts and space to check off the terms as they are called. Make a photocopy of this list for use in each game.
- **Prizes.** Some teachers like to award small prizes to the winners. This is optional; students can still have fun without them.

The Activity

- Provide each student with a bingo card.
- The caller calls out word parts randomly from the list. The caller checks off each word part as it is called.
- If the student's card has the word part that is called, the student draws an "X" through that space.
- The first player to get a row across, up and down, or diagonal calls out BINGO and may be the winner. Because some students will have similar cards, this adds to the excitement of the game.
- However, to be declared the winner, the player must be able to define each word part correctly.
- If an incorrect definition is given, the player is disqualified for that game and play continues until there is a winner.

Medical Word Part Bingo Caller's List

- *-AL* = pertaining to
- *-ALGIA* = pain and suffering
- *APPENDIC/O* = appendix
- *ARTERI/O* = artery
- *ARTHR/O* = joint
- *ATHER/O* = plaque or fatty substance
- *CARDI/O* = heart
- *CHONDR/O* = cartilage
- *COL/O* = colon
- *-DYNIA* = pain
- *DYS-* = difficult, painful or bad
- *-ECTOMY* = surgical removal
- *ENTER/O* = small intestine
- *GASTR/O* = stomach
- *-GRAPHY* = recording a picture
- *HEM/O* = relating to blood
- *HYPER-* = over, above, or increased
- *HYPO-* = below, under, or decreased
- *-IC* = pertaining to
- *-ITIS* = inflammation
- *LARYNG/O* = larynx
- *-MALACIA* = abnormal softening
- *-MEGALY* = large or enlargement
- *MYC/O* = fungus
- *MYEL/O* = spinal cord or bone marrow
- *MY/O* = muscle
- *-NECROSIS* = the death of tissue
- *NEPHR/O* = kidney
- *NEUR/O* = nerve
- *-OLOGIST* = specialist
- *-OLOGY* = study of
- *-OSIS* = a disease or abnormal condition
- *OSTE/O* = bone
- *OT/O* = ear
- *-OTOMY* = a surgical incision
- *-PATHY* = disease
- *PERI-* = surrounding
- *-PLASTY* = surgical repair
- *POLY-* = many
- *PY/O* = pus
- *RHIN/O* = nose
- *-RRHAGE* = abnormal or excessive flow
- *-RRHAPHY* = to suture or stitch
- *-RRHEA* = flow or discharge
- *-RRHEXIS* = rupture
- *-SCLEROSIS* = abnormal hardening
- *-SCOPY* = visual examination
- *-STENOSIS* = abnormal narrowing
- *SUB-* = under, less, or below
- *SUPRA-* = above, excessive, or beyond

MEDICAL WORD PART BINGO (1)

B	I	N	G	O
DYS-	-AL	-ECTOMY	-OSIS	-PLASTY
-ITIS	ARTHR/O	HYPER-	-OTOMY	-RRHEA
OSTE/O	-ALGIA	FREE	PERI-	-STENOSIS
GASTR/O	SUB-	-MALACIA	-RRHEXIS	MYEL/O
-RRHAPHY	CARDI/O-	-OLOGIST	-MEGALY	COL/O-

MEDICAL WORD PART BINGO (2)

B	I	N	G	O
HEM/O	-PATHY	OT/O	ARTERI/O	-SCOPY
-DYNIA	PY/O	NEUR/O	-IC	ENTER/O
DYS-	-OLOGY	FREE	SUPRA-	-GRAPHY
HYPO-	POLY-	MYC/O	ATHER/O	-OSIS
RHIN/O	CHONDR/O	-AL	PERI-	-ALGIA

MEDICAL WORD PART BINGO (3)

B	I	N	G	O
NEPHR/O	-OTOMY	-DYNIA	GASTR/O	-ITIS
-STENOSIS	-MEGALY	CARDI/O	PY/O	SUB-
HYPER-	-NECROSIS	FREE	OT/O	-MALACIA
LARYNG/O	ATHER/O	-ALGIA	-PLASTY	NEUR/O
-RRHAGE	-SCLEROSIS	COL/O	-ECTOMY	-PATHY

MEDICAL WORD PART BINGO (4)

B	I	N	G	O
OSTE/O	-RRHEA	ENTER/O	POLY-	-GRAPHY
-OLOGY	MY/O	APPENDIC/O	-IC	MYEL/O
-SCOPY	HYPER-	FREE	-PATHY	NEPHR/O
RHIN/O	DYS-	MYC/O	HYPO-	SUPRA-
HEM/O	-RRHAPHY	-OLOGIST	-ITIS	LARYNG/O

MEDICAL WORD PART BINGO (5)

B	I	N	G	O
-NECROSIS	PY/O	SUB-	-IC	LARYNG/O
-DYNIA	COL/O	ENTER/O	OT/O	-SCLEROSIS
-OSIS	GASTR/O	FREE	-RRHAPHY	MYC/O
MYEL/O	-ITIS	ARTHR/O	-MALACIA	-OLOGY
-SCOPY	CARDI/O	HEM/O	-MEGALY	PERI-

MEDICAL WORD PART BINGO (6)

B	I	N	G	O
-RRHEXIS	OSTE/O	NEUR/O	DYS-	-AL
-ALGIA	-OLOGIST	-GRAPHY	HYPER-	-RRHEA
RHIN/O	ATHER/O	FREE	-PLASTY	MY/O
-OTOMY	CHONDR/O	SUPRA-	-PATHY	OT/O
CARDI/O	GASTR/O	-IC	POLY-	-RRHAGE

MEDICAL WORD PART BINGO (7)

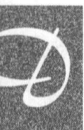

B	I	N	G	O
-AL	NEPHR/O	APPENDIC/O	-ITIS	-STENOSIS
LARYNG/O	ARTERI/O	-MALACIA	-OLOGY	-ALGIA
NEUR/O	-DYNIA	FREE	-PLASTY	-ECTOMY
CHONDR/O	MYC/O	-OTOMY	PERI-	-MEGALY
-RRHEA	HEM/O	-SCLEROSIS	DYS-	HYPO-

MEDICAL WORD PART BINGO (8)

B	I	N	G	O
-ALGIA	PY/O	OSTE/O	COL/O	HYPO-
GASTR/O	-AL	RHIN/O	ARTHR/O	-RRHEXIS
-NECROSIS	POLY-	FREE	MY/O	-PATHY
-GRAPHY	ENTER/O	-OLOGIST	NEPHR/O	-IC
MYEL/O	-SCOPY	-RRHAGE	OT/O	-RRHEA

MEDICAL WORD PART BINGO (9)

B	I	N	G	O
-OLOGY	NEPHR/O	COL/O	-RRHAPHY	-STENOSIS
ARTERI/O	PERI-	-NECROSIS	-ITIS	LARYNG/O
-PLASTY	-IC	FREE	MYC/O	APPENDIC/O
-OSIS	-DYNIA	CARDI/O	-RRHEXIS	-ECTOMY
SUPRA-	HYPER-	OSTE/O	HEM/O	ATHER/O

MEDICAL WORD PART BINGO (10)

B	I	N	G	O
-ALGIA	CARDI/O	-OLOGY	GASTR/O	RHIN/O
-MEGALY	-SCLEROSIS	CHONDR/O	ARTERI/O	HYPO-
SUB-	DYS-	FREE	-MALACIA	-RRHEA
OT/O	-PLASTY	ENTER/O	-IC	-NECROSIS
COL/O	MY/O	-ITIS	NEPHR/O	-ECTOMY

MEDICAL TERMINOLOGY BINGO CALLER'S LIST

MEDICAL TERMINOLOGY BINGO

B	I	N	G	O
		FREE		

Medical Word Part Bingo

SECTION

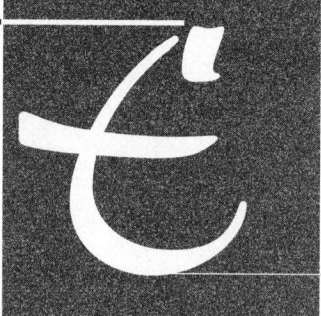

Jeopardy!®

Overview Of Jeopardy!®

Medical Word Part Jeopardy!

1. Grid for Medical Word Part Jeopardy!
2. Questions for Medical Word Part Jeopardy!

Body System Jeopardy!

3. Grid for Body System Jeopardy!
4. Questions for Skeletal System Jeopardy!
5. Questions for Muscular System Jeopardy!
6. Questions for Cardiovascular System Jeopardy!
7. Questions for Respiratory System Jeopardy!
8. Questions for Digestive System Jeopardy!
9. Questions for Urinary System Jeopardy!
10. Questions for Nervous System Jeopardy!
11. Questions for Integumentary System Jeopardy!
12. Questions for Reproductive Systems Jeopardy!

Purpose: This popular team activity is a medical terminology version of Jeopardy!®, the television quiz show. Version #1 is Word Part Jeopardy! Version #2 is Body System Jeopardy!

Advance Preparation

- **Grid.** Make an overhead transparency of the appropriate grid. During play, cross off categories as they are used. At the end of a game, wipe the grid clean ready for reuse.
- **Questions.** One set of questions has been supplied for each version. A form is also provided to help you create additional questions. An alternative to writing questions is to select the proper number of activity cards or flashcards relating to the version being played.
- **Show host.** The host, usually the teacher, asks the questions and marks off the categories as they are used.
- **Contestants.** The game can be played with three or four contestants who stand or are seated at the front of the room facing the audience. Contestants respond by raising their hands.
- **Scorekeeper.** One student is appointed as the scorekeeper. Scores are recorded on the board.
- **Judges.** Two students act as judges to decide who responded first and whether the response was correct.
- **Audience.** All other students are the audience. They must participate actively by applauding and trying to guess the right answers.

The Activity, Version #1

- The first contestant is selected randomly and is allowed to choose the first category and value.
- The host gives the "answer." The contestant responds with the appropriate "question." This format must be correct or the response is considered wrong.
- If the response is correct, points are added to that contestant's score. That contestant gets to select the next category and question value.
- If the response is not correct, points are subtracted from the contestant's score. Then the other contestants have an opportunity to answer the question.
- This round ends when all questions in all categories have been used.

The Activity, Version #2

- Play for this version is the same; however, the body systems grid and appropriate body system questions are used.

MEDICAL WORD PART JEOPARDY!

Prefixes	Combining Forms	Suffixes	Terms	Hodge Podge
100	100	100	100	100
200	200	200	200	200
300	300	300	300	300
400	400	400	400	400
500	500	500	500	500

QUESTIONS FOR MEDICAL WORD PART JEOPARDY!

	HOST	CONTESTANT
PREFIXES		
100	*PRE-*	What prefix means before?
200	*POST-*	What prefix means after?
300	*HYPO-*	What prefix means below, under, or decreased?
400	*POLY-*	What prefix means many?
500	*PERI-*	What prefix means surrounding?
COMBINING FORMS		
100	*CARDI/O*	What combining form means heart?
200	*NEUR/O*	What combining form means nerve?
300	*GASTR/O*	What combining form means stomach?
400	*MY/O*	What combining form means muscle?
500	*CYT/O*	What combining form means cell?
SUFFIXES		
100	*-ITIS*	What suffix means inflammation?
200	*-ECTOMY*	What suffix means surgical removal?
300	*-PLASTY*	What suffix means surgical repair?
400	*-RRHEA*	What suffix means flow or discharge?
500	*-RRHEXIS*	What suffix means rupture?
TERMS		
100	Tonsillitis	What term means inflammation of the tonsils?
200	Gastralgia	What term means pain in the stomach?
300	Renal	What term means pertaining to the kidney?
400	Appendectomy	What term means surgical removal of the appendix?
500	Myorrhaphy	What term means to suture a muscle?
HODGE PODGE		
100	*-MALACIA*	What suffix means abnormal softening?
200	*HYPER-*	What prefix means over, above, increased?
300	Natal	What root word means pertaining to birth?
400	*RHIN/O*	What combining form means nose?
500	A combining vowel	What is used when the suffix begins with a consonant?

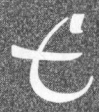

Use This Form to Develop Additional
QUESTIONS FOR MEDICAL WORD PART JEOPARDY!

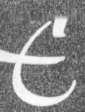

PREFIXES	HOST	CONTESTANT
100	_____	_____
200	_____	_____
300	_____	_____
400	_____	_____
500	_____	_____

COMBINING FORMS		
100	_____	_____
200	_____	_____
300	_____	_____
400	_____	_____
500	_____	_____

SUFFIXES		
100	_____	_____
200	_____	_____
300	_____	_____
400	_____	_____
500	_____	_____

TERMS		
100	_____	_____
200	_____	_____
300	_____	_____
400	_____	_____
500	_____	_____

HODGE PODGE		
100	_____	_____
200	_____	_____
300	_____	_____
400	_____	_____
500	_____	_____

BODY SYSTEM JEOPARDY!

Word Parts	Anatomy	Pathology	Procedures	Hodge Podge
100	100	100	100	100
200	200	200	200	200
300	300	300	300	300
400	400	400	400	400
500	500	500	500	500

QUESTIONS FOR SKELETAL SYSTEM JEOPARDY!

WORD PARTS	HOST	CONTESTANT
100	*ARTHR/O*	What combining form means joint?
200	*OSTE/O*	What combining form means bone?
300	*CHONDR/O*	What combining form means cartilage?
400	*MYEL/O*	What combining form means bone marrow and spinal cord?
500	*-DESIS*	What suffix means to bind or tie together?

ANATOMY

100	Mandible	What bone forms the lower jaw?
200	Foramen	What term means an opening in a bone?
300	Cranium	What bones encase the brain?
400	Manubrium	What is the upper portion of the sternum?
500	Carpals	What are the bones of the wrist?

PATHOLOGY

100	Arthralgia	What term means pain in a joint?
200	Chondromalacia	What term means abnormal softening of cartilage?
300	Osteoporosis	What term means the loss of bone density?
400	Lordosis	What term is also known as swayback?
500	Ankylosis	What term means the loss or absence of mobility in a joint?

PROCEDURES

100	Arthrotomy	What procedure is a surgical incision into a joint?
200	Arthroplasty	What procedure is the surgical replacement of a joint?
300	Bursectomy	What procedure is the surgical removal of a bursa?
400	Cranioplasty	What procedure is the surgical repair of the skull?
500	Arthrolysis	What procedure is surgical loosening of an ankylosed joint?

HODGE PODGE

100	Periosteum	What is the outer covering of bone?
200	Osteomalacia	What term means abnormal softening of bone?
300	Clavicle	What bone is also known as the collarbone?
400	Osteoarthritis	What term is also known as wear and tear arthritis?
500	Osteoclasis	What term means surgical fracture of a bone to correct a deformity?

QUESTIONS FOR MUSCULAR SYSTEM JEOPARDY!

WORD PARTS	HOST	CONTESTANT
100	*MY/O*	What combining form means muscle?
200	*-CELE*	What suffix means tumor, cyst, or hernia?
300	*-PLEGIA*	What suffix means paralysis?
400	*KINESI/O*	What combining form means movement?
500	*TAX/O*	What combining form means coordination?
ANATOMY		
100	Flexion	What term means decreasing the angle at a joint?
200	Abduction	What term means movement toward the midline?
300	Tendon	What attaches a muscle to bone or to another muscle?
400	Striated	What are also known as voluntary muscles?
500	Sphincter	What term means a ringlike muscle?
PATHOLOGY		
100	Myosclerosis	What term means abnormal hardening of muscle tissue?
200	Myalgia	What term means pain in a muscle?
300	Fasciitis	What term means inflammation of a fascia?
400	Epicondylitis	What term is also known as tennis elbow?
500	Singultus	What term is also known as hiccups?
PROCEDURES		
100	Myoplasty	What procedure is the surgical repair of a muscle?
200	Herniorrhaphy	What procedure is suturing of a hernia?
300	Fasciotomy	What procedure is a surgical incision of fascia?
400	Myectomy	What procedure is surgical removal of muscle?
500	Fasciorrhaphy	What procedure is suturing of torn fascia?
HODGE PODGE		
100	Spasm	What term is also known as a cramp?
200	Quadriplegia	What term means paralysis of all four extremities?
300	Myorrhexis	What term means rupture of a muscle?
400	Claudication	What term means lameness or limping?
500	Torticollis	What term is also known as wryneck?

QUESTIONS FOR CARDIOVASCULAR SYSTEM JEOPARDY!

	WORD PARTS	HOST	CONTESTANT
	100	*CARDI/O*	What combining form means heart?
	200	*ARTERI/O*	What combining form means artery?
	300	*LEUK/O*	What combining form means white?
	400	*-RRHAGE*	What suffix means bursting forth?
	500	*PHLEB/O*	What combining form means vein?
ANATOMY			
	100	Aorta	What is the largest of the arteries?
	200	Erythrocytes	What term means red blood cells?
	300	Endocardium	What term means the lining of the heart?
	400	Venae cavae	What large veins return blood to the heart?
	500	Atria	What are the upper chambers of the heart?
PATHOLOGY			
	100	Cardiomegaly	What term means abnormal enlargement of the heart?
	200	Aneurysm	What terms means a balloon-like enlargement of an artery?
	300	Myocardial infarction	What term is also known as a heart attack?
	400	Phlebitis	What term means inflammation of a vein?
	500	Embolus	What is a foreign object circulating in the blood?
PROCEDURES			
	100	Angiography	What procedure is a radiographic study of blood vessels?
	200	Valvuloplasty	What procedure is the surgical repair of a heart valve?
	300	Coronary bypass	What procedure improves the blood supply to the heart muscle?
	400	Defibrillation	What procedure uses electrical shock to restore the heart's normal rhythm?
	500	Electrocardiography	What test measures electrical activity of the myocardium?
HODGE PODGE			
	100	Cardiorrhexis	What term means rupture of the heart?
	200	Palpitation	What term means a pounding, racing heart?
	300	Cholesterol	What fatty substance builds up on the walls of arteries?
	400	Hemostasis	What term means to control bleeding?
	500	Balloon angioplasty	What procedure opens a partially blocked artery?

QUESTIONS FOR RESPIRATORY SYSTEM JEOPARDY!

WORD PARTS	HOST	CONTESTANT
100	*LARYNG/O*	What combining form means larynx?
200	*TRACHE/O*	What combining form means trachea?
300	*CYAN/O*	What combining form means blue?
400	*PHON/O*	What combining form means sound or voice?
500	*-PNEA*	What suffix means breathing?
ANATOMY		
100	Diaphragm	What muscle separates the chest and abdomen?
200	Epiglottis	What acts as a lid so food does not enter the lungs?
300	Trachea	What is commonly known as the windpipe?
400	Sinus	What is an air-filled cavity within a bone?
500	Pleura	What membranes encase the lungs?
PATHOLOGY		
100	Laryngitis	What term means inflammation of the larynx?
200	Pneumorrhagia	What term means bleeding from the lungs?
300	Epistaxis	What term is also known as a nosebleed?
400	Anthracosis	What term is also known as black lung disease?
500	Pertussis	What term is also known as whooping cough?
PROCEDURES		
100	Laryngectomy	What procedure is the surgical removal of the larynx?
200	Pharyngoplasty	What procedure is the surgical repair of the pharynx?
300	Bronchodilator	What medication expands the passages into the lungs?
400	Tracheotomy	What emergency procedure is an incision into the trachea?
500	Thoracotomy	What procedure is a surgical incision into the wall of the chest?
HODGE PODGE		
100	Laryngoplegia	What term means paralysis of the larynx?
200	Olfactory	What are the receptors for the sense of smell?
300	Hyperventilation	What term means abnormally rapid deep breathing?
400	Asphyxiation	What term is also known as suffocation?
500	Sputum	What is phlegm called when ejected through the mouth?

QUESTIONS FOR DIGESTIVE SYSTEM JEOPARDY!

WORD PARTS	HOST	CONTESTANT
100	*GASTR/O*	What combining form means stomach?
200	*ENTER/O*	What combining form means small intestine?
300	*COL/O*	What combining form means large intestine?
400	*HEPAT/O*	What combining form means Liver?
500	*CHOL/E*	What combining form means bile or gall?

ANATOMY		
100	Pancreas	What organ produces pancreatic juices?
200	Duodenum	What is the first part of the small intestine?
300	Anus	What is the lower opening of the digestive tract?
400	Gallbladder	Where is bile stored until needed?
500	Glycogen	What is the stored form of glucose?

PATHOLOGY		
100	Colitis	What term means inflammation of the colon?
200	Hepatomegaly	What term means abnormal enlargement of the liver?
300	Gastrorrhea	What term means excessive flow of gastric juices?
400	Cholecystitis	What term means inflammation of the gallbladder?
500	Cirrhosis	What is a progressive degenerative disease of the liver?

PROCEDURES		
100	Appendectomy	What procedure is the surgical removal of the appendix?
200	Proctoplasty	What procedure is the surgical repair of the rectum?
300	Colostomy	What procedure is the creation of an opening between the colon and the surface of the body?
400	Ileectomy	What procedure is the surgical removal of the ileum?
500	Gastropexy	What procedure is the surgical fixation of the stomach?

HODGE PODGE		
100	Peristalsis	What action is responsible for the movement of food?
200	Digestion	What process converts foods into nutrients for body use?
300	*PEPS/O*	What combining form means to digest or digestion?
400	Enzymes	What chemicals are responsible for breaking down food?
500	Jaundice	What term means a yellow discoloration of the skin?

QUESTIONS FOR URINARY SYSTEM JEOPARDY!

WORD PARTS	HOST	CONTESTANT
100	*NEPHR/O*	What combining form means kidney?
200	*URIN/O*	What combining form means pertaining to urine?
300	*-URIA*	What suffix means urination or relating to urine?
400	*LITH/O*	What combining form means stone or calculus?
500	*-ECTASIS*	What suffix means enlargement or stretching?

ANATOMY		
100	Nephron	What is the structural unit of the kidney?
200	Ureter	What carries urine from the kidney to the bladder?
300	Renal pelvis	Where is urine collected before it enters the ureters?
400	Urethra	What carries urine from the bladder to outside the body?
500	Meatus	What is the external opening of a passage?

PATHOLOGY		
100	Cystitis	What term means inflammation of the bladder?
200	Oliguria	What term means scanty urination?
300	Dysuria	What term means difficult or painful urination?
400	Nephroptosis	What term means prolapse of the kidney?
500	Ureterectasis	What term means distention of a ureter?

PROCEDURES		
100	Nephrectomy	What procedure is the surgical removal of a kidney?
200	Cystoscopy	What procedure is the visual examination of the bladder?
300	Urethrorrhaphy	What procedure means to suture the urethra?
400	Lithotripsy	What procedure destroys a stone using sound waves?
500	Cystopexy	What procedure is the surgical fixation of the bladder?

HODGE PODGE		
100	Polyuria	What term means excessive urination?
200	Dialysis	What procedure is the removal of waste products from the blood of patients whose kidneys no longer function?
300	Enuresis	What term is also known as bed-wetting?
400	Pyelitis	What term means inflammation of the renal pelvis?
500	Nephropyosis	What term means suppuration formation in the kidney?

QUESTIONS FOR NERVOUS SYSTEM JEOPARDY!

WORD PARTS	HOST	CONTESTANT
100	*NEUR/O*	What combining form means nerve?
200	*MYEL/O*	What combining form means spinal fluid?
300	*ENCEPHAL/O*	What combining form means brain?
400	*POLI/O*	What combining form means gray matter of nerves?
500	*-ESTHESIA*	What suffix means sensation or feeling?
ANATOMY		
100	Cerebellum	What is the second largest part of the brain?
200	Afferent neuron	What type of neuron carriers messages to the brain?
300	Meninges	What connective tissues enclose the brain?
400	Myelin sheath	What is the protective covering over some nerves?
500	Synapse	What is the space between two neurons?
PATHOLOGY		
100	Polyneuritis	What term means inflammation affecting many nerves?
200	Encephalitis	What term means inflammation of the brain?
300	Meningitis	What term means inflammation of the meninges?
400	Syncope	What term means the brief loss of consciousness?
500	Bell's palsy	What is paralysis of the facial nerve?
PROCEDURES		
100	Neuroplasty	What procedure is the surgical repair of a nerve?
200	Neurectomy	What procedure is the surgical removal of a nerve?
300	Neurotomy	What procedure is a surgical incision into a nerve?
400	Neurorrhaphy	What term means to suture the ends of a severed nerve?
500	Encephalography	What is an x-ray study of the brain?
HODGE PODGE		
100	Myelitis	What term means inflammation of the spinal cord?
200	Concussion	What term means violent shaking of the brain?
300	Sciatica	What term means inflammation of the sciatic nerve?
400	Hydrocephalus	What term means abnormally increased spinal fluid in the brain?
500	Radiculitis	What term means inflammation of the root of a spinal nerve?

QUESTIONS FOR INTEGUMENTARY SYSTEM JEOPARDY!

WORD PARTS	HOST	CONTESTANT
100	*CUTANE/O*	What combining form means skin?
200	*SEB/O*	What combining form means sebum?
300	*HIDR/O*	What combining form means sweat?
400	*UNGU/O*	What combining form means nail?
500	*MELAN/O*	What combining form means black or dark?
ANATOMY		
100	Epidermis	What is the outermost layer of the skin?
200	Lipocytes	What are also known as fat cells?
300	Keratin	What fibrous protein makes up epidermis hair, and nails?
400	Eponychium	What term is also known as the cuticle of the nail?
500	Hidrosis	What term means sweat?
PATHOLOGY		
100	Hirsutism	What term means abnormal hairiness?
200	Pruritus	What term means itching?
300	Xeroderma	What term means excessively dry skin?
400	Alopecia	What term means a complete lack of hair?
500	Ecchymosis	What term is also known as a bruise?
PROCEDURES		
100	Biopsy	What procedure is the removal of a piece of tissue for examination?
200	Rhinoplasty	What procedure is the surgical repair of the nose?
300	Liposuction	What procedure is the surgical removal of fat?
400	Debridement	What procedure is the removal of dirt or foreign objects from a wound?
500	Rhytidectomy	What procedure is the surgical removal of wrinkles?
HODGE PODGE		
100	*GANGRIN/O*	What combining form means gangrene or eating sore?
200	Urticaria	What term is also known as hives?
300	Bulla	What term means a large vesicle or blister?
400	Onychomycosis	What term means a fungus infection of the nail?
500	Rhinophyma	What term means overgrowth of skin and oil glands of the nose?

QUESTIONS FOR REPRODUCTIVE SYSTEMS JEOPARDY!

WORD PARTS	HOST	CONTESTANT
100	*HYSTER/O*	What combining form means uterus?
200	*COLP/O*	What combining form means vagina?
300	*METR/O*	What combining form means uterus?
400	*OOPHOR/O*	What combining form means ovary?
500	*ORCHID/O*	What combining form means testes?

ANATOMY		
100	Scrotum	What sac encloses and supports the testicles?
200	Ova	What are the female gametes or eggs?
300	Prepuce	What term is also known as the foreskin?
400	Perineum	What region is between the vaginal orifice and the anus?
500	Endometrium	What is the lining of the uterus?

PATHOLOGY		
100	Vaginocele	What term means a hernia of the vagina?
200	Metrorrhea	What term means an abnormal uterine discharge?
300	Pruritus vulvae	What term means itching of the external female genitalia?
400	Dysmenorrhea	What term means a difficult or painful monthly flow?
500	Ovariorrhexis	What term means rupture of an ovary?

PROCEDURES		
100	Parturition	What is the act of giving birth?
200	Circumcision	What procedure is the surgical removal of the foreskin?
300	Episiorrhaphy	What procedure is suturing an episiotomy?
400	Vasectomy	What procedure is sterilization in the male?
500	Colporrhaphy	What procedure means suturing the vagina?

HODGE PODGE		
100	Lactation	What term means the process of secreting milk?
200	Prostatorrhea	What term means a discharge from the prostate gland?
300	Preeclampsia	What term is also known as toxemia of pregnancy?
400	Pyosalpinx	What term means pus in the fallopian tube?
500	Mittelschmerz	What term means pain between menstrual periods?

Use This Form to Develop Additional
QUESTIONS FOR BODY SYSTEM JEOPARDY!

WORD PARTS	HOST	CONTESTANT
100		
200		
300		
400		
500		
ANATOMY		
100		
200		
300		
400		
500		
PATHOLOGY		
100		
200		
300		
400		
500		
PROCEDURES		
100		
200		
300		
400		
500		
HODGE PODGE		
100		
200		
300		
400		
500		

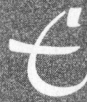

Jeopardy!®

SECTION F

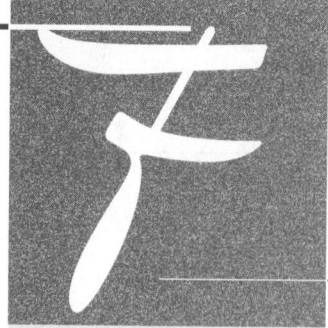

Crossword Puzzles

Overview of Crossword Puzzles

1. Medical Word Part Crossword Puzzle
2. Medical Specialties Crossword Puzzle
3. The Skeletal System Crossword Puzzle
4. The Muscular System Crossword Puzzle
5. The Cardiovascular System Crossword Puzzle
6. The Respiratory System Crossword Puzzle
7. The Digestive System Crossword Puzzle
8. The Urinary System Crossword Puzzle
9. The Nervous System Crossword Puzzle
10. The Integumentary System Crossword Puzzle
11. The Reproductive Systems Crossword Puzzle
12. General Medical Terminology Crossword Puzzle

MEDICAL WORD PART CROSSWORD PUZZLE

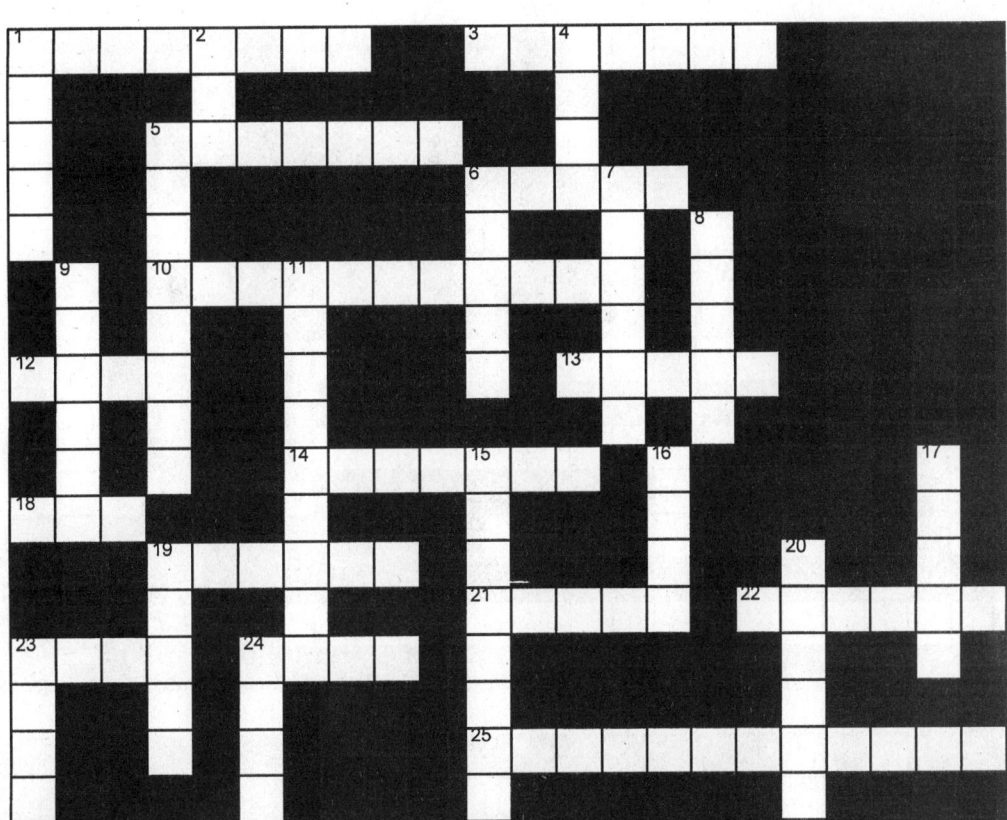

MEDICAL WORD PART CROSSWORD PUZZLE CLUE LIST

Across

1. Suffix meaning abnormal narrowing.
3. Suffix meaning to rupture.
5. Pertaining to the heart.
6. Suffix meaning the study of.
10. Inflammation of the tonsils.
12. Suffix meaning inflammation.
13. Suffix meaning flow or discharge.
14. Suffix meaning to suture.
18. Prefix meaning difficult, painful, or bad.
19. Suffix meaning surgical repair.
21. Combining form meaning nerve.
22. Combining form meaning heart.
23. Suffix meaning after.
24. Suffix meaning a disease or abnormal condition.
25. Surgical removal of the appendix.
26. Prefix meaning many.

Down

1. Suffix meaning direct visual examination.
2. Suffix meaning tumor or neoplasm.
4. Prefix meaning below, under, or decreased.
5. Suffix meaning surgical puncture to remove fluid.
6. Combining form meaning scanty or few.
7. Combining form meaning stomach.
8. Prefix meaning over, above, or increased.
9. Suffix meaning surgical removal.
11. Suffix meaning abnormal hardening.
15. Time and events before birth.
16. Combining form meaning colon.
17. Suffix meaning pain.
19. Suffix meaning disease.
20. Suffix meaning abnormal softening.
23. Prefix meaning surrounding.
24. Suffix meaning a surgical incision.

MEDICAL SPECIALTIES CROSSWORD PUZZLE

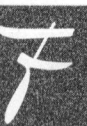

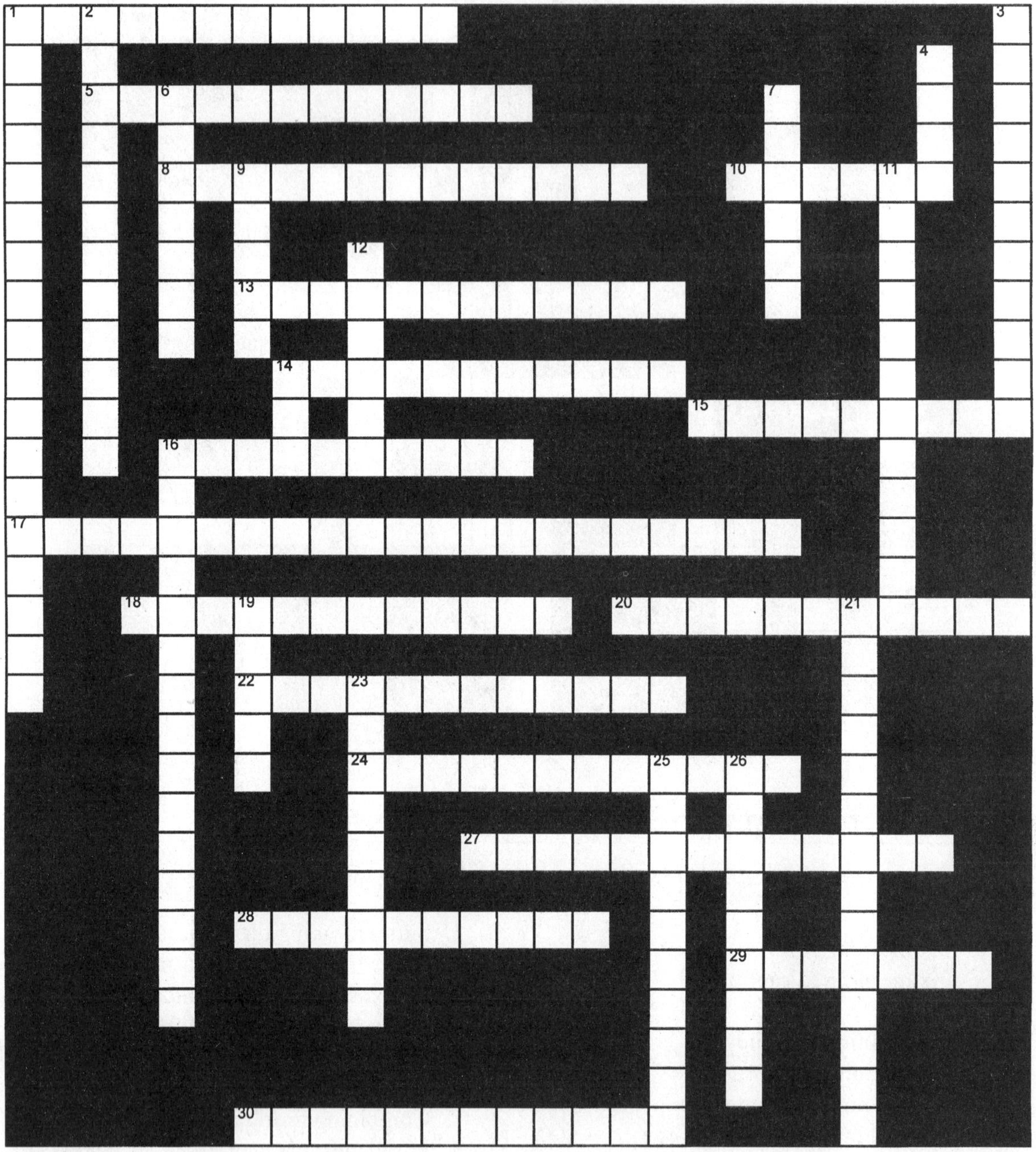

MEDICAL SPECIALTIES CROSSWORD PUZZLE CLUE LIST

Across

1. A specialist in disorders of the female reproductive system.
5. A specialist in diseases and disorders of children.
8. A specialist in the care of the newborn.
10. Combining form meaning female.
13. A specialist in disorders of the blood and bloodforming tissues.
14. A specialist in measuring visual acuity.
15. Study of the nerves.
16. A specialist in malignant disorders such as tumors and cancer.
17. A specialist in the treatment of the ears, nose, and throat.
18. A specialist in manipulative treatment of disorders originating from misalignment of the spine.
20. A specialist, other than a physician, in the administration of anesthesia.
22. A specialist in the study of the immune system.
24. A specialist in providing medical care relating to pregnancy and childbirth.
27. A specialist in disorders of the skin.
28. A specialist in disorders of the feet.
29. Combining form meaning old.
30. A specialist in disorders of the rectum and anus.

Down

1. A specialist in disorders of the stomach and intestines.
2. A specialist in disorders of the kidneys.
3. The study of the process and problems of aging.
4. Combining form meaning cancer.
6. A specialist in disorders of the teeth and tissues of the mouth.
7. Combining form meaning mind.
9. Combining form meaning straight or normal.
11. A specialist in disorders of the cardiovascular system.
12. Combining form meaning stomach.
14. Combining form meaning ear.
16. A specialist in diseases and disorders of the eye.
19. Combining form meaning nose.
21. A specialist in the study of outbreaks of disease within a population group.
23. A specialist in disorders of the urinary system.
25. A specialist in the study of cells.
26. A specialist in altered immunologic reactivity.

THE SKELETAL SYSTEM CROSSWORD PUZZLE

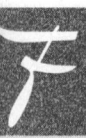

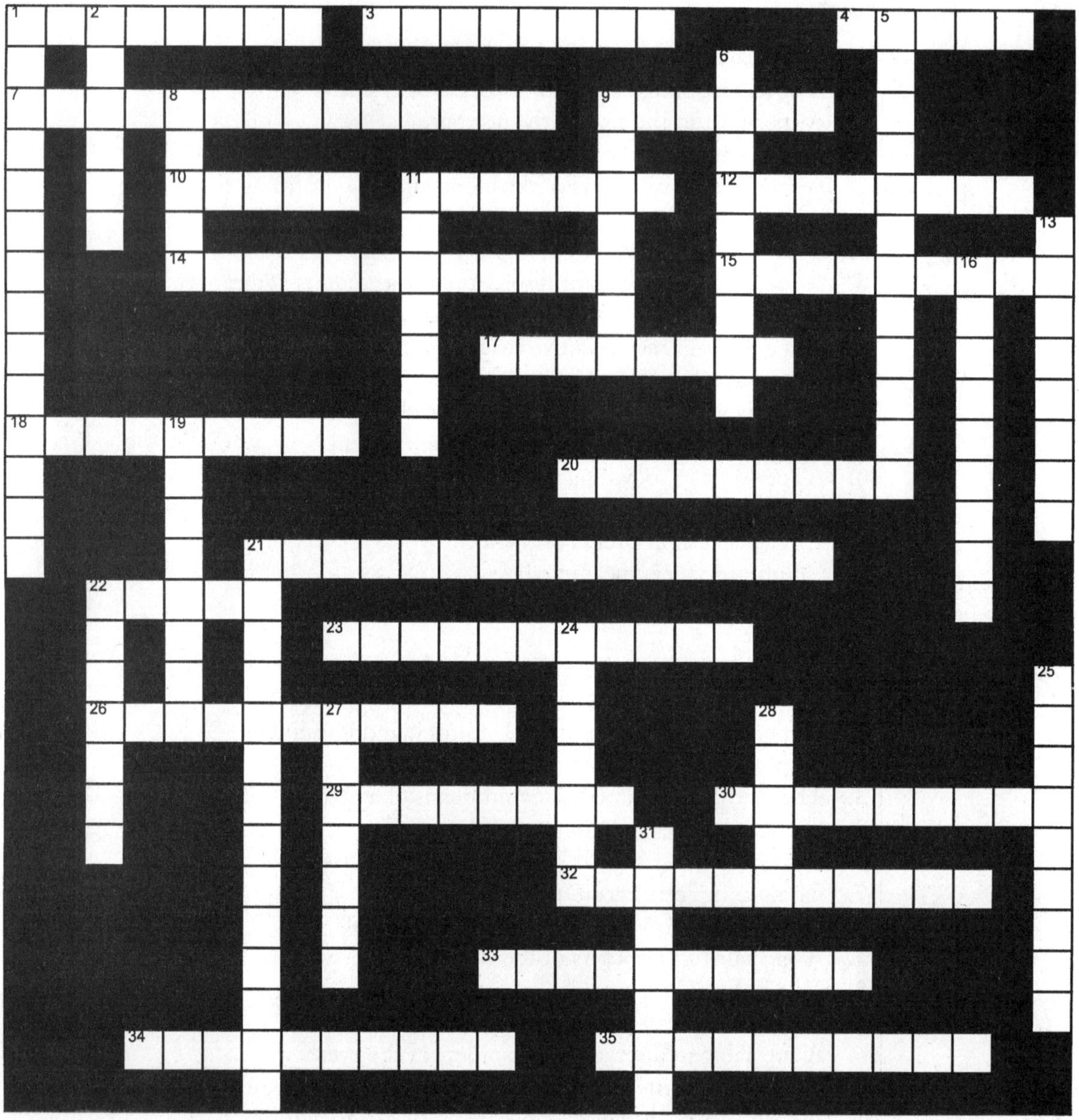

THE SKELETAL SYSTEM CROSSWORD PUZZLE CLUE LIST

Across

1. Also known as the collarbone.
3. Inflammation of bone.
4. Combining form meaning rib.
7. Wear and tear arthritis.
9. Also known as the tailbone.
10. Also known as the skin bone.
11. Combining form meaning cartilage.
12. Also known as swayback.
14. Abnormal softening of bone.
15. A surgical incision into a bone.
17. Inflammation of a bursa.
18. Loss or absence of mobility in a joint.
20. A benign growth on a bone.
21. Abnormal stiffening of a joint.
22. The upper leg bone.
23. Any disease of a joint.
26. Surgical loosening of an ankylosed joint.
29. The lower jaw.
30. Bones that make up the spinal column.
32. Visual examination of the interior of a joint.
33. Pain in a joint.
34. Tissue surrounding bone.
35. Surgical removal of a bursa.

Down

1. Abnormal softening of cartilage.
2. Combining form meaning joint.
5. Abnormal thinning of bone associated with aging.
6. Any degenerative condition of the spine.
8. Combining form meaning bone.
9. Bones of the wrist.
11. Also known as the skull.
13. Also known as humpback.
16. Also known as the funny bone.
19. Connective tissue bands that join the articulating ends of bones.
21. Surgical puncture to remove fluid from a joint.
22. An opening in a bone through which blood vessels, nerves, and ligaments pass.
24. Also known as the kneecap.
25. Pain associated with any disorder of bone.
27. Also known as low back pain.
28. Combining form meaning bone marrow and spinal cord.
31. Also known as the breastbone.

THE MUSCULAR SYSTEM CROSSWORD PUZZLE

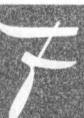

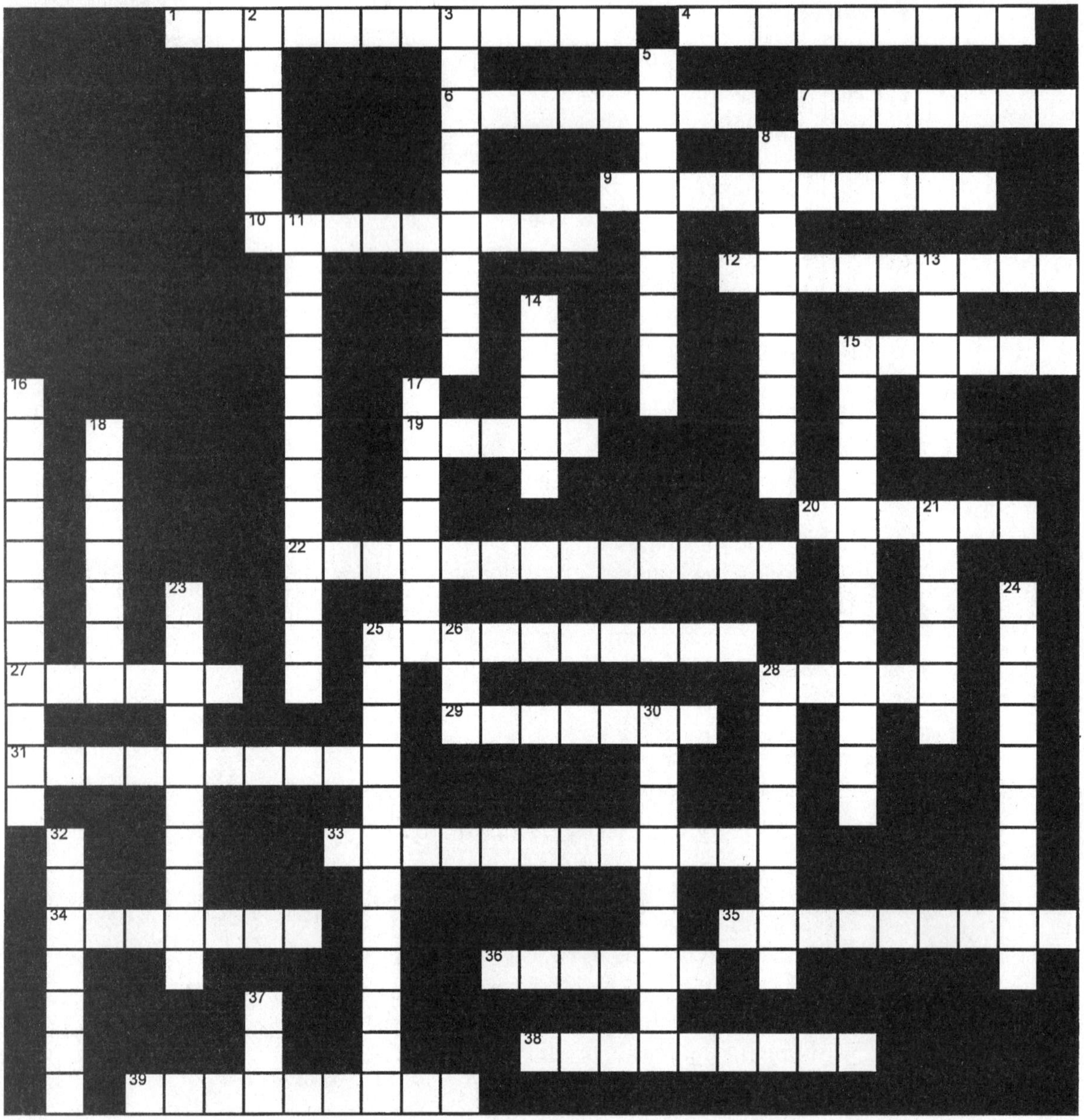

THE MUSCULAR SYSTEM CROSSWORD PUZZLE CLUE LIST

Across

1. Lameness or limping.
4. Inflammation of a fascia.
6. Difficulty in controlling voluntary movement.
7. Weakness and wasting away caused by disuse of a muscle.
9. Total paralysis of one side of the body.
10. Movement away from the midline.
12. Also known as hiccups.
15. Combining form meaning fascia.
19. Suffix meaning pain.
20. Muscle of the anterior upper arm.
22. Also known as tennis elbow.
25. Paralysis of both legs and the lower part of the body.
27. Connective tissue that attaches a muscle to bone.
28. Sudden, violent, involuntary contraction of a muscle.
29. Muscle tenderness or pain.
31. To suture a muscle wound.
33. Abnormally increased motor function or activity.
34. A muscle slanted at an angle.
35. To free a tendon from adhesions.
36. The place where a muscle begins.
38. Turns downward or backward.
39. To suture the end of a tendon to bone.

Down

2. Inability to coordinate the muscles in the execution of voluntary movement.
3. Movement toward the midline.
5. To increase the angle in a limb.
8. A ringlike muscle.
11. Extreme slowness in movement.
13. Suffix meaning to set free.
14. Suffix meaning to bind or tie together.
15. Surgical repair of a fascia.
16. Surgical removal of fascia.
17. Suffix meaning abnormal softening.
18. Decreases the angle in a limb.
21. Suffix meaning surgical removal.
23. The rupture of a muscle.
24. Abnormal softening of a muscle.
25. Inflammation of several voluntary muscles simultaneously.
26. Abbreviation describing type of movements made possible by muscles.
28. Also known as voluntary muscles.
30. The place where a muscle ends.
32. Protrusion of a muscle through its ruptured sheath.
37. Combining form meaning muscle.

THE CARDIOVASCULAR SYSTEM CROSSWORD PUZZLE

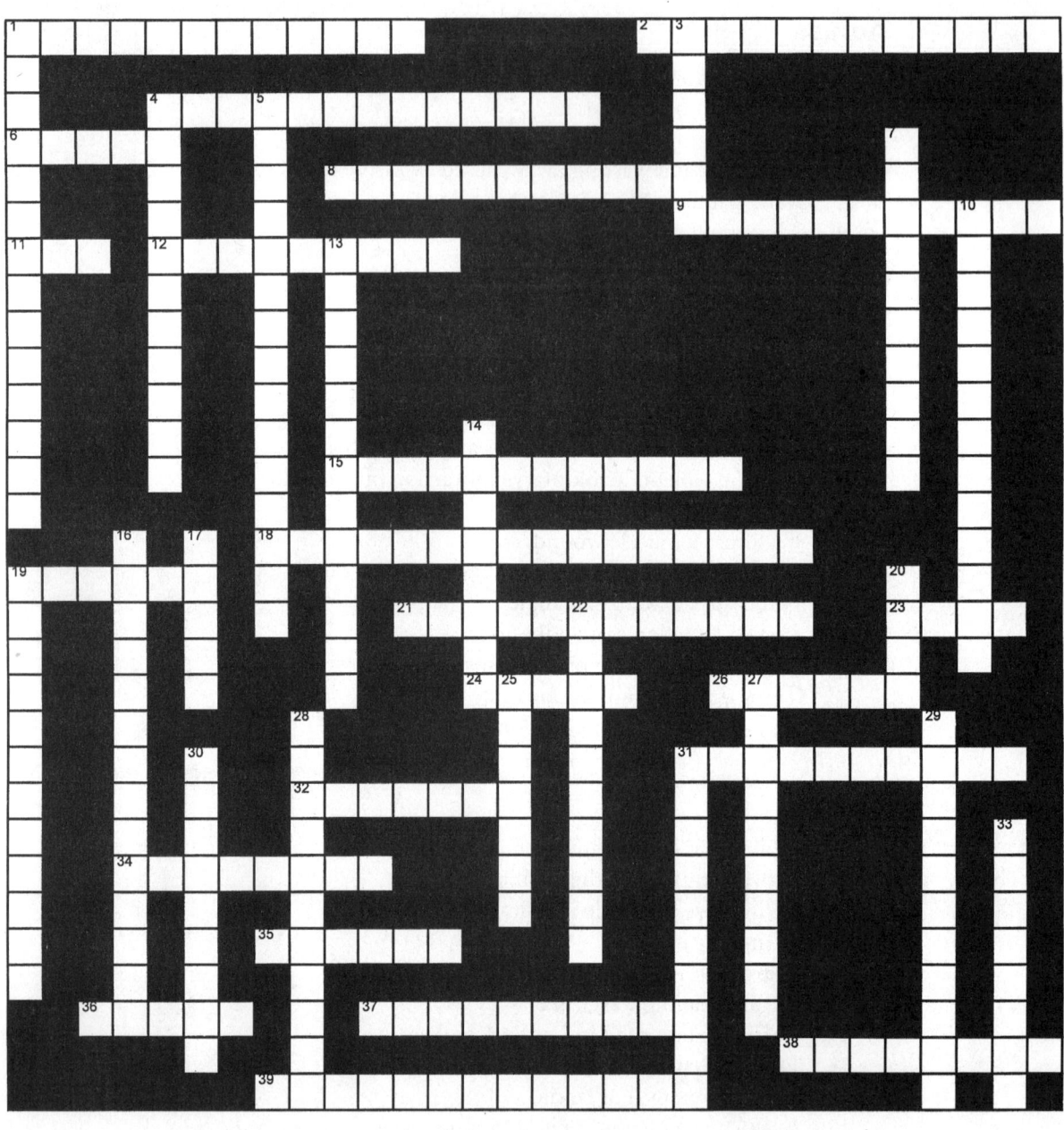

THE CARDIOVASCULAR SYSTEM CROSSWORD PUZZLE CLUE LIST

Across

1. Inflammation of the inner layer of the heart.
2. Enlargement of the heart.
4. Surgical repair of a heart valve.
6. Upper chambers of the heart.
8. A pounding racing heart beat.
9. A radiographic study of blood vessels.
11. Abbreviation for electrocardiogram.
12. Any abnormal or pathologic disorder of the blood.
15. Red blood cells.
18. Inflammation of a vein with a thrombus.
19. Combining form meaning plaque or fatty substance.
21. Rapid, random, and ineffective contractions of the heart.
23. Suffix meaning blood or blood condition.
24. Plasma with the clotting proteins removed.
26. Combining form meaning vein.
31. The loss of a large amount of blood in a short time.
32. Combining form meaning artery.
34. Localized balloon-like enlargement of an artery.
35. Combining form meaning heart.
36. Combining form meaning blood and lymph vessels.
37. Inflammatory condition of a heart valve.
38. Inflammation of the heart.
39. Rupture of the heart.

Down

1. Surgical removal of plaque from clogged arteries.
3. Spasmodic, choking, or suffocating pain.
4. A drug that expands the blood vessels.
5. A drug the narrows the blood vessels.
7. Irregularity of the heartbeat.
10. Inflammation involving several arteries.
13. The tissue death of the walls of blood vessels.
14. A blood clot attached to the interior wall of a blood vessel.
16. Restoration of the heart's normal rhythm by electrical shock.
17. Main trunk of the arterial system.
19. The surgical removal of part of an artery.
20. Combining form meaning vein.
22. White blood cells.
25. A foreign object circulating in the blood.
27. A benign tumor made up of newly formed blood vessels.
28. An abnormally slow heartbeat.
29. An abnormally fast heartbeat.
30. Inflammation of a vein.
31. To control bleeding.
33. A malignancy characterized by a progressive increase of abnormal leukocytes.

THE RESPIRATORY SYSTEM CROSSWORD PUZZLE

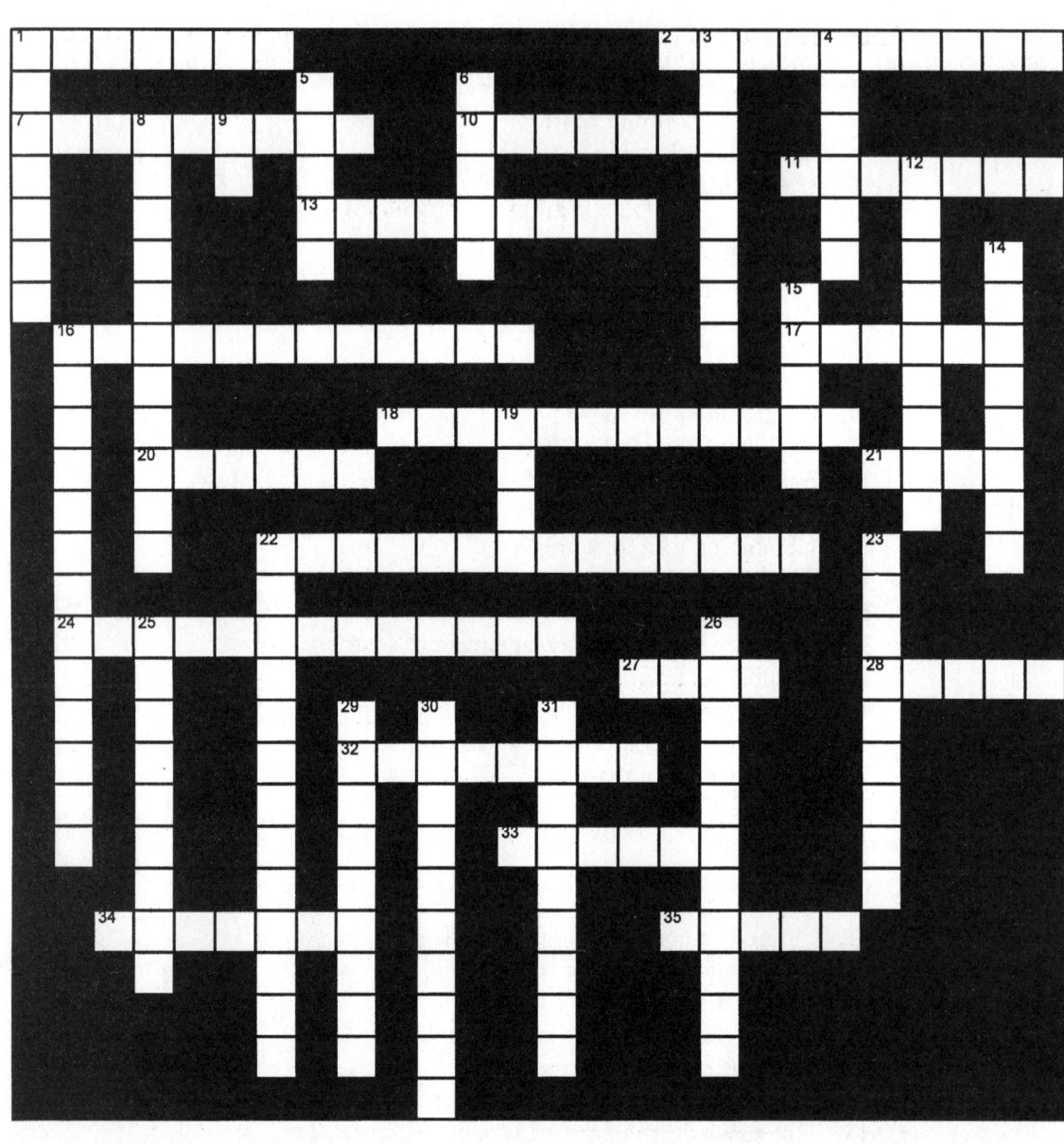

THE RESPIRATORY SYSTEM CROSSWORD PUZZLE CLUE LIST

Across

1. Also known as the windpipe.
2. Acts as lid to prevent food from entering lungs.
7. Sense of smell.
10. Loss of the ability to produce normal speech sounds.
11. Difficult or labored breathing.
13 Muscle separating the check and abdomen.
16. Surgical creation of an artificial opening into the trachea.
17. Membranes surrounding each lung.
18. Excessive flow of mucus from the bronchi.
20. Phlegm ejected through the mouth.
21. Abbreviation for sudden infant death syndrome.
22. Bleeding from the bronchi.
24. Bleeding from the lungs.
27. Suffix meaning breathing.
28. Combining form meaning sound or voice.
32. Inflammation of the pleura in the thoracic cavity.
33. Specialized membrane lining the nose.
34. Accumulation of pus in the pleural or other body cavity.
35. Air-filled cavity within a bone.

Down

1. Combining form meaning thorax.
3. Combining form meaning pharynx or throat.
4. Also known as the voice box.
5. Prefix meaning slow.
6. Prefix meaning rapid.
8. Also known as black lung disease.
9. Abbreviation for disease caused by *Mycobacterium tuberculosis*.
12. Also known as whooping cough.
14. Blue color.
15. The absence of spontaneous respiration.
16. Surgical repair of the trachea.
19. Combining form meaning nose.
22. Paralysis of the walls of the bronchi.
23. Any voice impairment such as hoarseness.
25. Progressive loss of lung function caused by enlargement of the alveoli.
26. Region between the lungs.
29. Also known as a nosebleed.
30. An accumulation of blood in the pleural cavity.
31. Inflammation of a sinus.

THE DIGESTIVE SYSTEM CROSSWORD PUZZLE

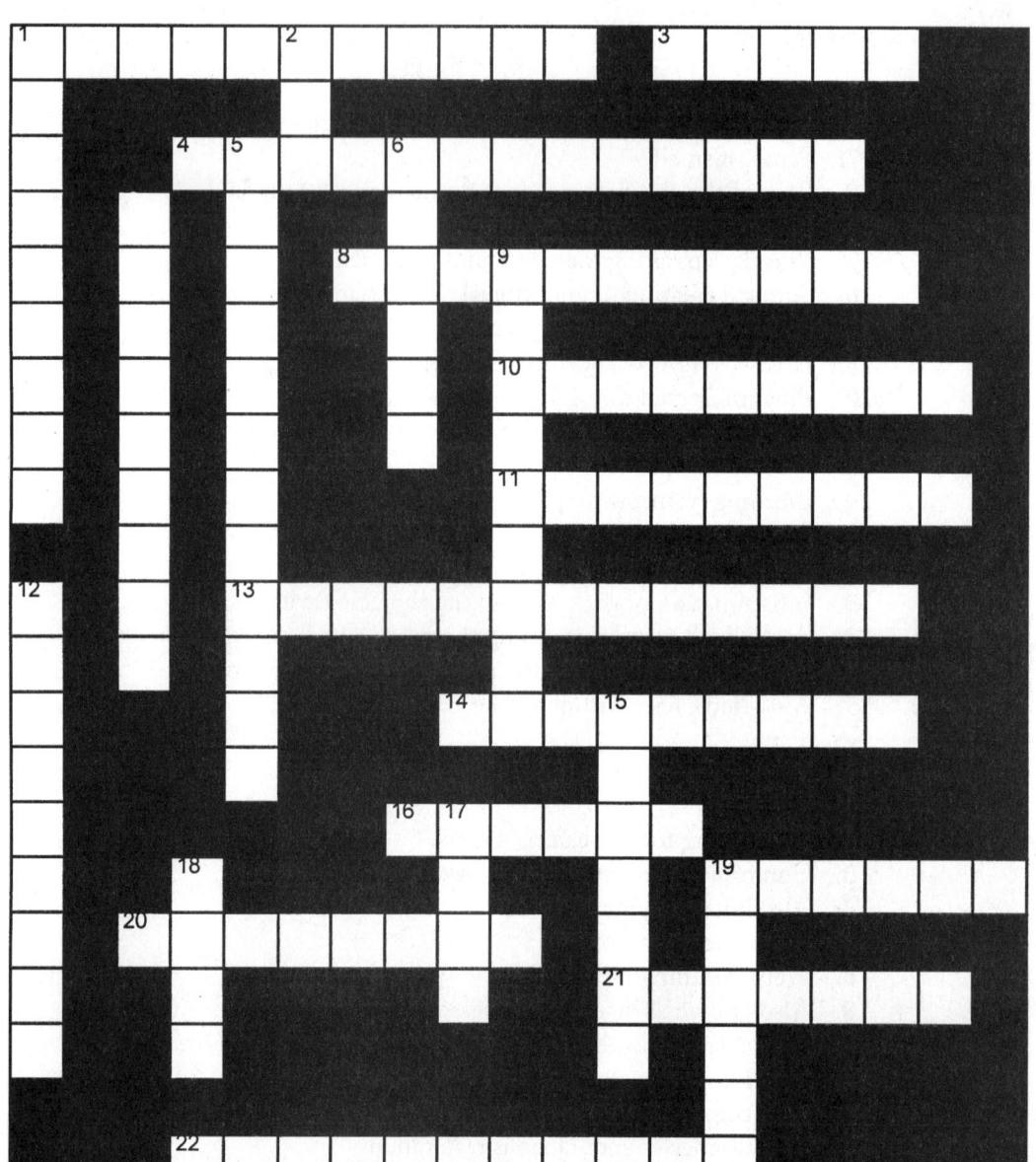

THE DIGESTIVE SYSTEM CROSSWORD PUZZLE CLUE LIST

Across

1. Surgical creation of an opening into the stomach.
3. Solid body wastes expelled through the rectum.
4. Inflammation of the gallbladder.
8. Wavelike motion that moves food through the intestines.
10. Also known as the gullet.
11. Surgical creation of an opening between the colon and the body surface.
13. Rupture of the stomach.
14. Also known as indigestion.
16. Combining form meaning stomach.
19. Combining form meaning small intestine.
20. Twisting of the intestine on itself that causes an obstruction.
21. Inflammation of the ileum.
22. Vomiting blood.

Down

1. Inflammation of the stomach.
2. Combining form meaning mouth.
5. Abnormal enlargement of the liver.
6. A substances that causes vomiting.
7. Inflammation of the liver.
9. Surgical removal of all, or part of, the ileum.
12. Surgical repair of the anus.
15. Also known as heartburn.
17. Lower opening of the digestive tract.
18. Combining form meaning large intestine.
19. Also known as vomiting

THE URINARY SYSTEM CROSSWORD PUZZLE

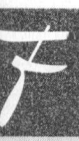

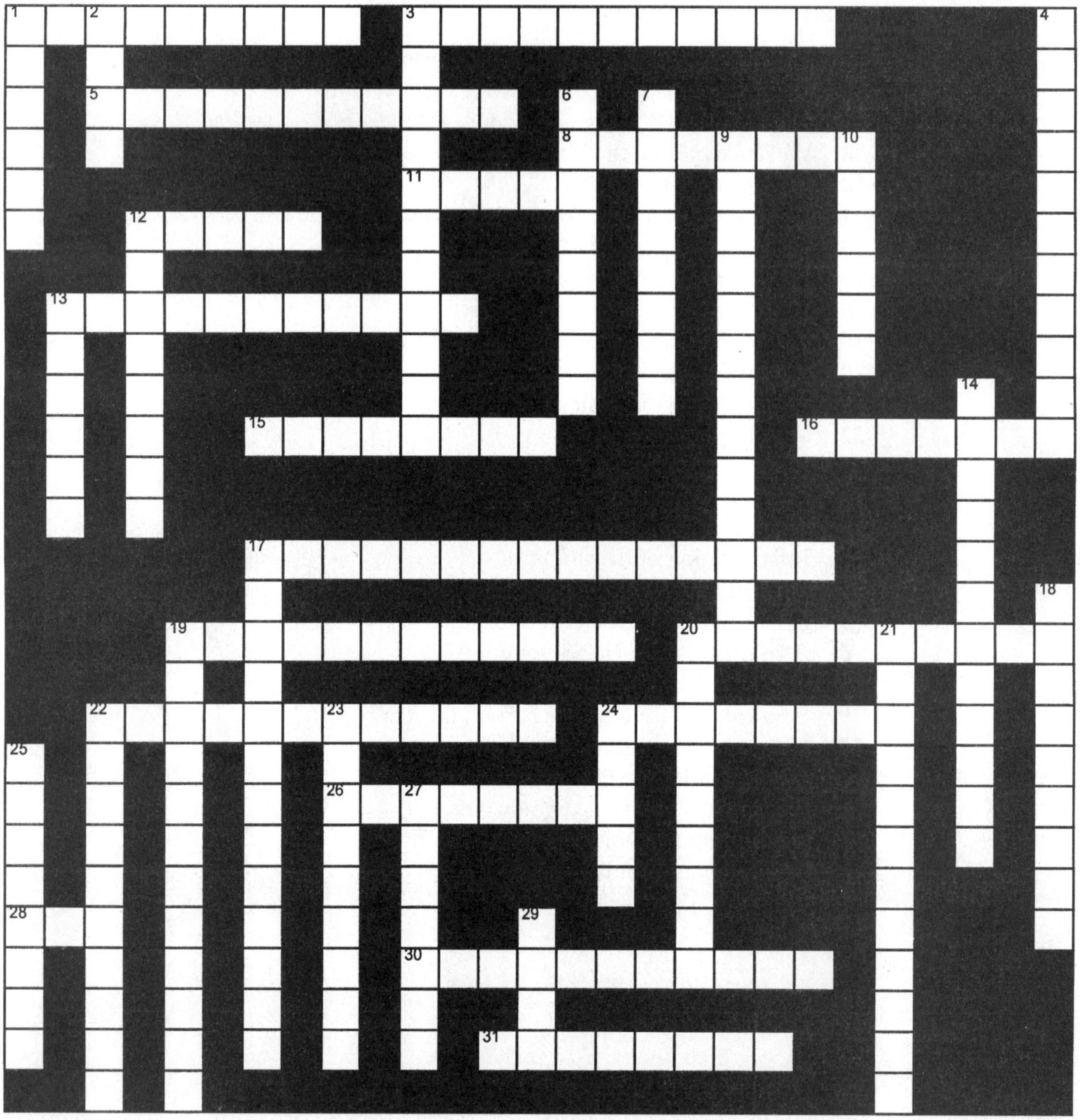

THE URINARY SYSTEM CROSSWORD PUZZLE CLUE LIST

Across

1. Inflammation of the kidneys.
3. Freeing a kidney from adhesions.
5. Destruction of a kidney stone using sound waves.
8. Scanty urination.
11. Pertaining to the kidneys.
12. Combining form meaning renal pelvis.
13. A stone lodged in the ureter.
15. Removal of waste products from the blood of patients whose kidneys no longer function.
16. Difficult or painful urination.
17. The presence of stones in the kidney.
19. Distention of a kidney.
20. Surgical removal of the bladder.
22. The formation or presence of pus in the kidney.
24. Inflammation of the bladder.
26. Also known as bed-wetting.
28. Combining form meaning urine.
30. Distention of the ureter due to blockage.
31. A tube inserted into a body cavity to remove or insert fluid.

Down

1. Combining form meaning kidney.
2. Prefix meaning many.
3. Surgical removal of a kidney.
4. Pain in the urethra.
6. Excessive urination.
7. Increased excretion of urine.
9. Surgical repair of a ureter.
10. Complete suppression of urine formation by the kidneys.
12. Inflammation of the renal pelvis.
13. Tube that carries urine from the kidney to the bladder.
14. Abnormal discharge from the urethra.
17. Abnormal softening of the kidneys.
18. Surgical fixation of the bladder to the abdominal wall.
19. Also known as floating kidney.
20. Hernia of the bladder through the vaginal wall.
21. Bleeding from the bladder.
22. Also known as a kidney stone.
23. A surgical incision into the renal pelvis.
24. Combining form meaning bladder.
25. Excessive urination during the night.
27. Tube that carries urine from the bladder to the exterior of the body.
29. Suffix meaning urination, urine.

THE NERVOUS SYSTEM CROSSWORD PUZZLE

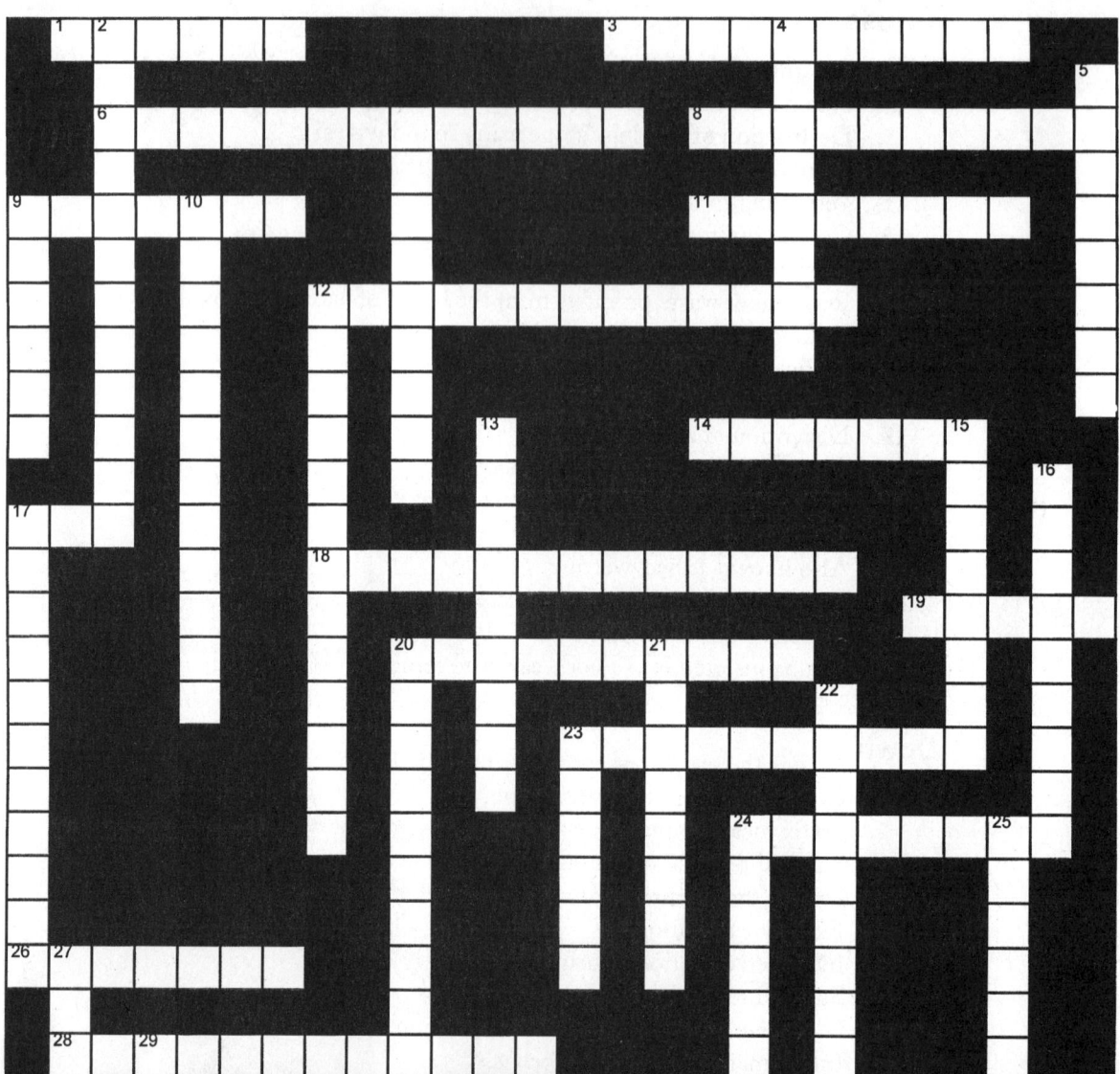

THE NERVOUS SYSTEM CROSSWORD PUZZLE CLUE LIST

Across

1. Suffix meaning speak or speech.
3. Inflammation of the meninges.
6. Viral infection of the spinal cord. Also known as polio.
8. Surgical removal of a nerve.
9. Also known as lockjaw.
11. Regional anesthesia during childbirth.
12. Excessive sensitivity to stimuli.
14. Also known as fainting.
17. Abbreviation for cerebral spinal fluid.
18. Congenital gap in the skull with herniation of brain substance.
19. Combining form meaning nerve.
20. Uncontrolled contractions of the skeletal muscles.
23. Uncontrollable seizures of drowsiness and sleep.
24. Inflammation of the sciatic nerve.
26. Memory loss.
28. Inflammation of the brain.
30. An automatic, involuntary response to change.
31. Refers to one in a coma.

Down

2. Part of the brain that controls vital body functions.
4. Inflammation of a nerve.
5. Inflammation of the spinal cord.
7. Combining form meaning brain.
9. Involuntary shaking or trembling.
10. Suturing of a nerve.
12. Abnormally increased amount of cerebrospinal fluid within the brain.
13. An impairment of speech due to a brain lesion.
15. A group of neurologic disorders characterized by recurrent episodes of seizures.
16. Pain in a nerve or nerves.
17. Pain in the head.
20. Also known as sleepwalking.
21. Uppermost and least protected layer of the brain.
22. Protrusion of the membranes of the brain through a defect in the skull.
23. The basic cell of the nervous system.
24. Also known as a convulsion.
25. Combining form meaning head.
27. Combining form meaning spinal cord and bone marrow.
29. Abbreviation. Also known as a stroke.

THE INTEGUMENTARY SYSTEM CROSSWORD PUZZLE

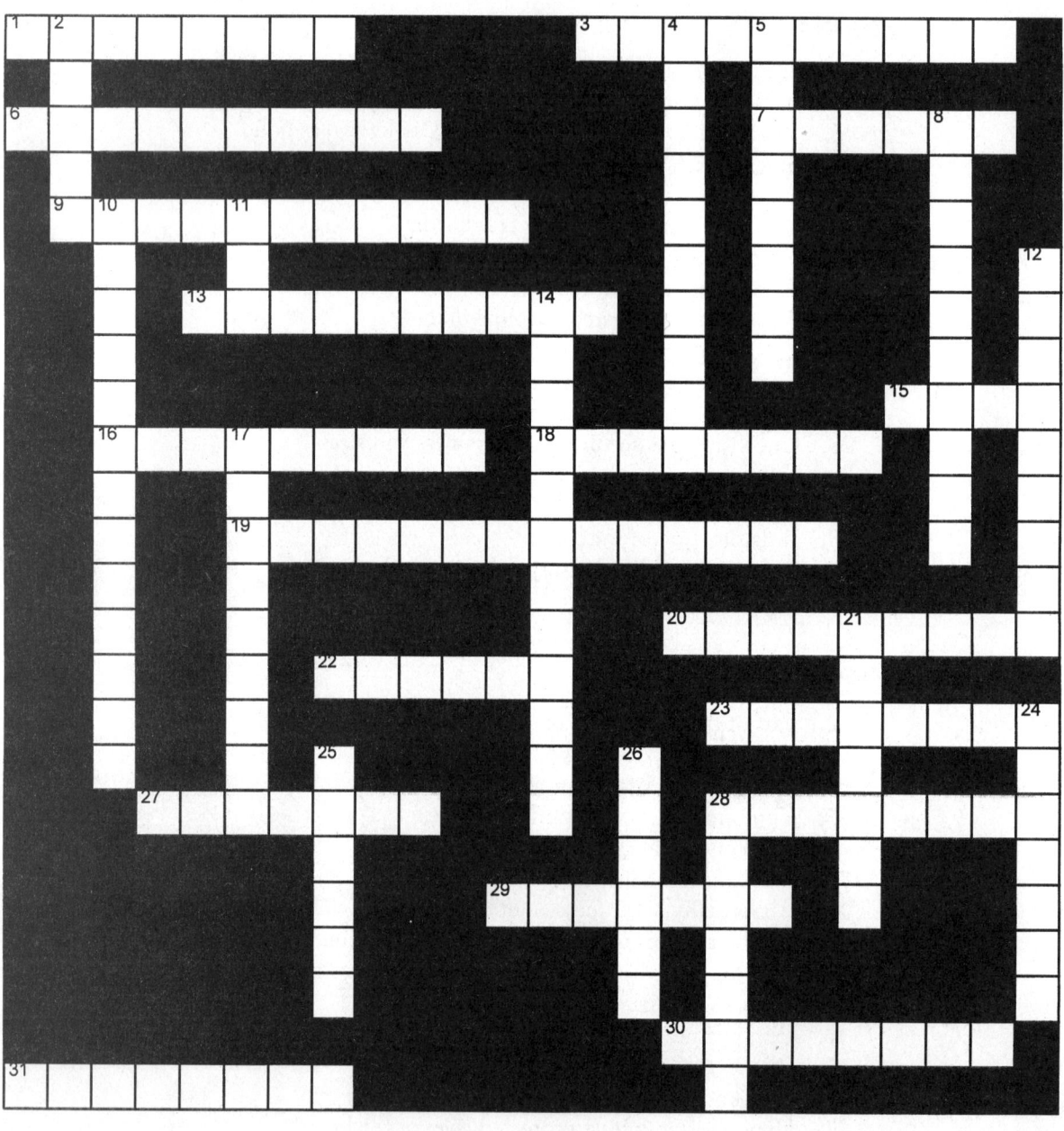

THE INTEGUMENTARY SYSTEM CROSSWORD PUZZLE CLUE LIST

Across

1. Producing or containing pus.
3. Inflammation of the skin.
6. Also known as a bruise.
7. Combining form meaning nail.
9. Surgical repair of the nose.
13. A torn or jagged wound.
15. Combining form meaning fat.
16. Excessive hairiness.
18. A normal healed scar.
19. Also known as a lid lift.
20. Excessively dry skin.
22. A benign tumor made up of mature fat cells.
23. Itching.
27. A localized collection of pus.
28. Also known as skin cancer.
29. Also known as a blister.
30. Production and excretion of sweat.
31. Tissue death.

Down

2. An open sore or erosion of the skin.
4. Also known as bulbous nose.
5. Also known as baldness.
8. A benign tumor of newly formed blood vessels.
10. Excessive sweating.
11. Suffix meaning tumor.
12. Excessive flow of sebum.
14. Also known as nail-biting.
17. Glands that lubricate the skin.
21. Combining form meaning skin.
24. Infestation with the itch mite.
25. An abnormally raised scar.
26. A pathologic tissue change due to disease or injury.
28. Pigment that determines skin color.

THE REPRODUCTIVE SYSTEMS CROSSWORD PUZZLE

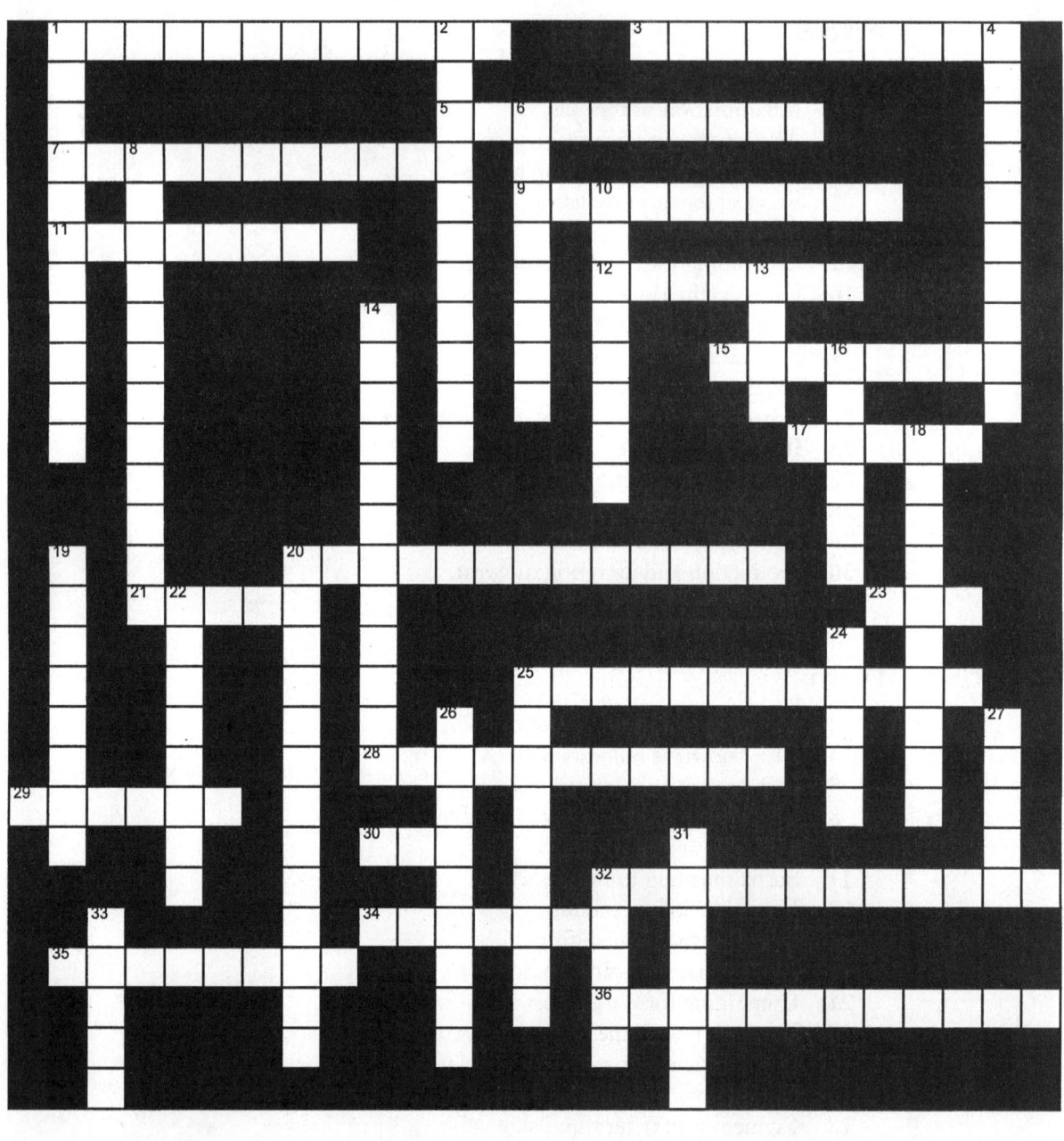

THE REPRODUCTIVE SYSTEMS CROSSWORD PUZZLE CLUE LIST

Across

1. Surgical removal of the uterus.
3. Abnormal uterine discharge.
5. Surgical removal of a breast.
7. Inner lining of the uterus.
9. Surgical removal of part of a breast.
11. One male organ that produces sperm.
12. External sac that encloses and supports the testes.
15. Male gland surrounding the neck of the bladder.
17. Ejaculatory fluid that contains sperm.
20. Time and events surrounding menopause.
21. Score to evaluate a newborn's physical status.
23. Abbreviation for pelvic inflammatory disease.
25. Surgical repair of the vagina.
28. Absence of sperm in the semen.
29. Combining form meaning vagina.
30. Common name for Papanicolaou test.
32. Surgical removal of the foreskin of the penis.
34. Combining form meaning ovary.
35. The beginning of menstruation.
36. A woman during her first pregnancy.

Down

1. Enlargement or overgrowth of tissue.
2. Radiographic examination of the breast.
4. Absence of the monthly menstrual flow.
6. Combining form meaning tube.
8. Difficult or painful monthly flow.
10. Inflammation of a breast.
13. Abbreviation for transurethral resection.
14. A woman who has never been pregnant.
16. Combining form meaning male gamete.
18. A surgical incision to facilitate delivery.
19. Delivery of a child through an incision in the maternal abdominal and uterine wall.
20. An abnormal flow of prostatic fluid.
22. Also known as the afterbirth.
24. Combining form meaning breast.
25. Male sterilization procedure.
26. Surgical fixation of the vagina to a surrounding structure.
27. Combining form meaning breast.
31. Combining form meaning testes.
32. Combining form meaning vagina.
33. Combining form meaning uterus.

GENERAL MEDICAL TERMINOLOGY CROSSWORD PUZZLE

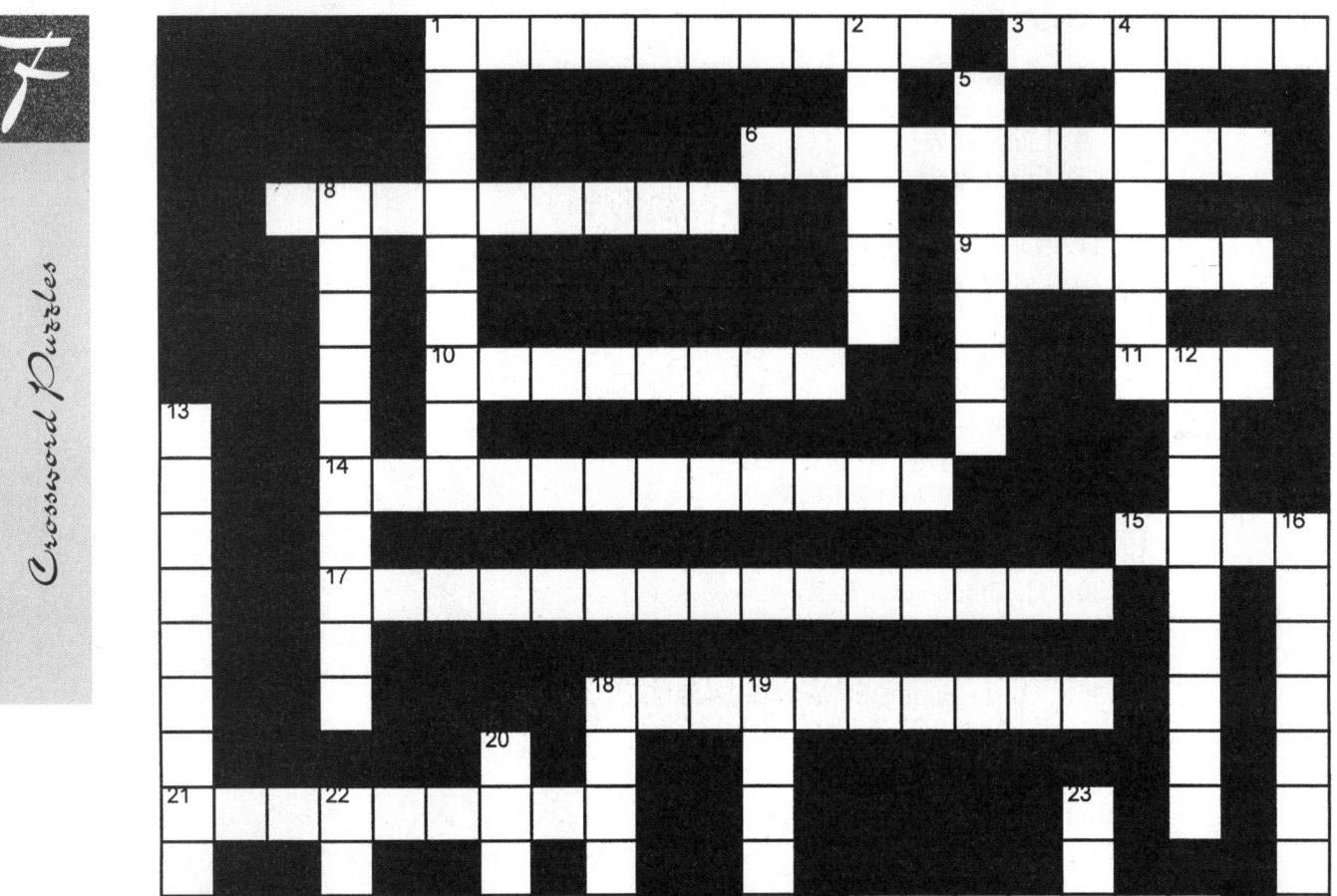

GENERAL MEDICAL TERMINOLOGY CROSSWORD PUZZLE CLUE LIST

Across

1. A substance that eases the severity of a disease but does not cure it.
3. Wound or injury.
6. Administration of medication by injection.
7. The determination of the cause of a disease.
9. A disease, structure, or procedure named for the person who discovered it first.
10. A set of signs and symptoms that occur together.
11. Abbreviation for magnetic resonance imaging.
14. Listening to sounds within the body.
15. Evidence of disease that can be observed by the patient and others.
17. A preoccupation with fears of having a serious disease.
18. The patient's following of a prescribed regimen.
21. An examination procedure using the hands.
24. To determine the priority of need and proper place of treatment.
25. A disease or symptom that lasts a long time.
26. Drug administration through the unbroken skin.
27. Abbreviation for a method of pain control using electronic impulses.
28. Evidence that can be observed only by the patient.

Down

1. A forecast of the probable outcome of a disorder.
2. Possessing masculine traits.
4. A word formed from the initial letters or letters of the major parts of a compound term.
5. The ongoing presence of a disease within a population, group, or area.
8. An illness without known cause.
12. The temporary disappearance of the symptoms of a chronic or malignant disease.
13. An instrument used for visual examination of the interior of an organ.
16. A hospital-acquired infection.
18. The surgical removal of fluid for diagnostic purposes.
19. Also known as venipuncture.
20. Pertaining to a virus.
22. A disease-producing organism.
23. Occurring over a large geographic area, possibly worldwide.

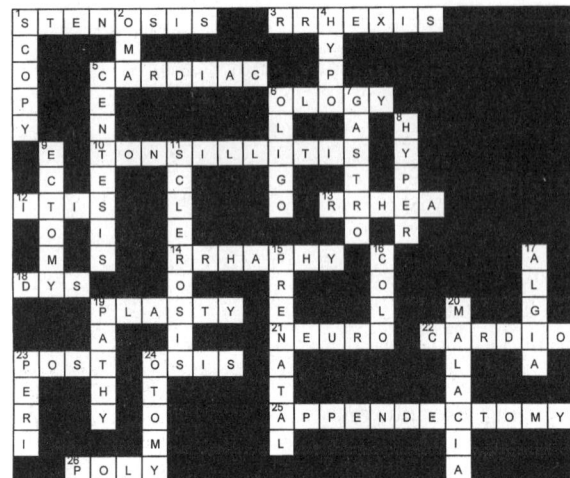

Medical Word Part
Crossword Puzzle Solution

Medical Specialties
Crossword Puzzle Solution

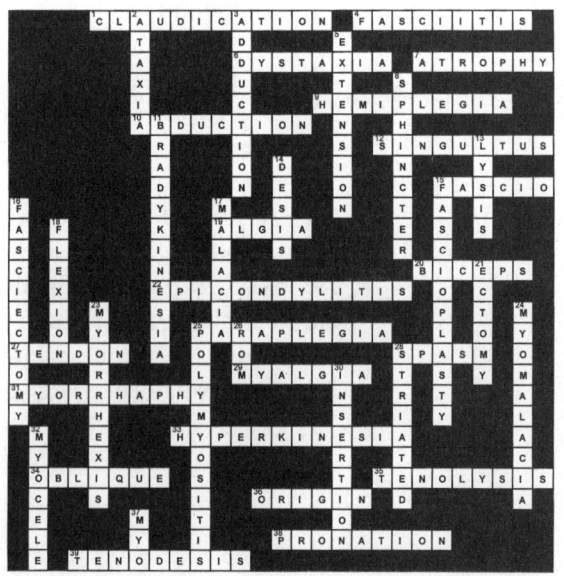

The Skeletal System
Crossword Puzzle Solution

The Muscular System
Crossword Puzzle solution

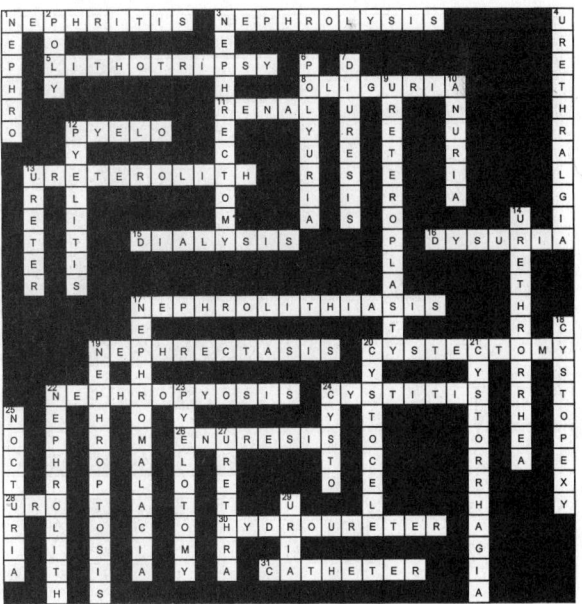

The Cardiovascular System
Crossword Puzzle Solution

The Respiratory System
Crossword Puzzle Solution

The Digestive System
Crossword Puzzle Solution

The Urinary System
Crossword Puzzle Solution

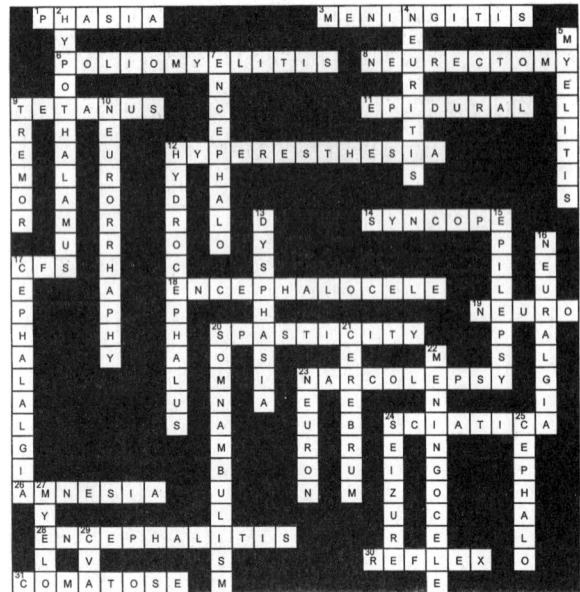

The Nerve System
Crossword Puzzle Solution

The Integumentary System
Crossword Puzzle Solution

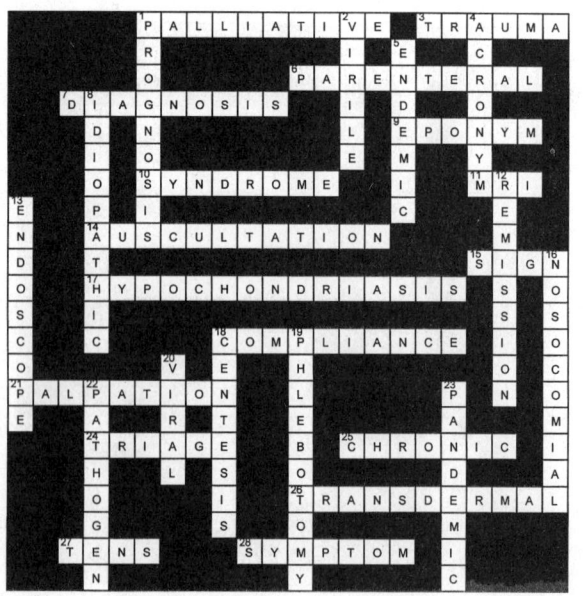

The Reproductive Systems
Crossword Puzzle solution

General Medical Terminology
Crossword Puzzle solution

SECTION G

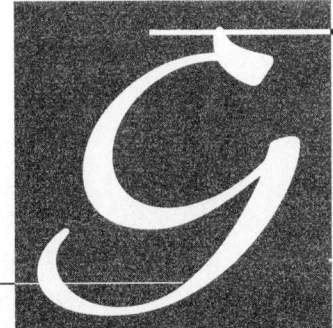

Activity Cards

Overview of Activity Cards

1. Medical Specialty Activity Cards
2. The Skeletal System Activity Cards
3. The Muscular System Activity Cards
4. The Cardiovascular System Activity Cards
5. The Immune System and Oncology Activity Cards
6. The Respiratory System Activity Cards
7. The Digestive System Activity Cards
8. The Urinary System Activity Cards
9. The Nervous System Activity Cards
10. Eyes and Ears Activity Cards
11. The Integumentary System Activity Cards
12. The Endocrine System Activity Cards
13. The Male Reproductive System Activity Cards
14. Pregnancy and Childbirth Activity Cards
15. The Female Reproductive System Activity Cards
16. Examination Terminology Activity Cards
17. Endoscopic Examination Activity Cards
18. General Medical Terminology Activity Cards

MEDICAL SPECIALTY ACTIVITY CARDS

Allergist (**AL**-er-jist)	**Epidemiologist** (**ep**-ih-**dee**-me-**OL**-oh-jist)
Anesthesiologist (**an**-es-**thee**-zee-**OL**-oh-jist)	**Gastroenterologist** (**gas**-troh-**en**-ter-**OL**-oh-jist)
Anesthetist (ah-**NES**-theh-tist)	**Gerontologist** (**jer**-on-**TOL**-oh-jist)
Cardiologist (**kar**-dee-**OL**-oh-jist)	**Gynecologist** (**guy**-neh-**KOL**-oh-jist)
Chiropractor (**KYE**-roh-**prack**-tor)	**Hematologist** (**hem**-ah-**TOL**-oh-jist)
Dermatologist (**der**-mah-**TOL**-oh-jist)	**Immunologist** (**im**-you-**NOL**-oh-jist)
Endocrinologist (**en**-doh-krih-**NOL**-oh-jist)	**Neonatologist** (**nee**-oh-nay-**TOL**-oh-jist)

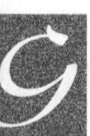

A specialist in the study of outbreaks of disease within a population group.	A specialist in diagnosing and treating conditions of altered immunologic reactivity.
A specialist in diagnosing and treating diseases and disorders of the stomach and intestines.	A physician who specializes in administering anesthetic agents before and during surgery.
A specialist in diagnosing and treating diseases, disorders, and problems associated with aging.	A person trained in administering anesthesia but who is not necessarily a physician.
A specialist in diagnosing and treating diseases and disorders of the female reproductive system.	A specialist in diagnosing and treating abnormalities, diseases, and disorders of the heart.
A specialist in diagnosing and treating diseases and disorders of the blood and blood-forming tissues.	A specialist in manipulative treatment of disorders originating from misalignment of the spine.
A specialist in the study of the immune system.	A specialist in diagnosing and treating disorders of the skin.
A specialist in diagnosing and treating disorders of the newborn.	A specialist in diagnosing and treating diseases and malfunctions of the glands of internal secretion.

Nephrologist (neh-**FROL**-oh-jist)	**Pathologist** (pah-**THOL**-oh-jist)
Neurologist (new-**ROL**-oh-jist)	**Pediatrician** (**pee**-dee-ah-**TRISH**-un)
Obstetrician (**ob**-steh-**TRISH**-un)	**Podiatrist** (poh-**DYE**-ah-trist)
Oncologist (ong-**KOL**-oh-jist)	**Proctologist** (prock-**TOL**-oh-jist)
Ophthalmologist (ahf-thal-**MOL**-oh-jist)	**Psychiatrist** (sigh-**KYE**-ah-trist)
Optometrist (op-**TOM**-eh-trist)	**Psychologist** (sigh-**KOL**-oh-jist)
Orthopedist (**or**-thoh-**PEE**-dist)	**Urologist** (you-**ROL**-oh-jist)

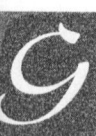

A specialist who performs the laboratory analysis of tissue samples to confirm or establish a diagnosis.	A specialist in diagnosing and treating diseases and disorders of the kidneys.
A specialist in diagnosing, treating, and preventing disorders and diseases of children.	A specialist in diagnosing and treating diseases and disorders of the nervous system.
A specialist in diagnosing, treating, and correcting disorders of the foot.	A specialist in providing medical care to women during pregnancy, childbirth, and immediately thereafter.
A specialist in disorders of the rectum and anus.	A specialist in diagnosing and treating malignant disorders such as tumors and cancer.
A physician who specializes in diagnosing and treating chemical dependencies, emotional problems, and mental illness.	A specialist in diagnosing and treating diseases and disorders of the eye.
A specialist, other than a physician, who evaluates and treats emotional problems.	A specialist in measuring the accuracy of vision to determine if corrective lenses or eyeglasses are needed.
A specialist in diagnosing and treating diseases and disorders of the urinary system of females and the genitourinary system of males.	A specialist in diagnosing and treating diseases and disorders involving the bones, joints, and muscles.

THE SKELETAL SYSTEM ACTIVITY CARDS

Ankylosis (ang-kih-**LOH**-sis)	**Bursectomy** (ber-**SECK**-toh-me)
Arthritis (ar-**THRIGH**-tis)	**Bursitis** (ber-**SIGH**-tis)
Arthrodesis (**ar**-throh-**DEE**-sis)	**Chondromalacia** (**kon**-droh-mah-**LAY**-she-ah)
Arthrography (ar-**THROG**-rah-fee)	**Chondroplasty** (**KON**-droh-**plas**-tee)
Arthrolysis (ar-**THROL**-ih-sis)	**Craniotomy** (**kray**-nee-**OT**-oh-me)
Arthroplasty (**AR**-throh-**plas**-tee)	**Exostosis** (**eck**-sos-**TOH**-sis)
Arthrosclerosis (**ar**-throh-skleh-**ROH**-sis)	**Kyphosis** (kye-**FOH**-sis)

Activity Cards

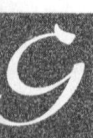

The surgical removal of a bursa.	The loss or absence of mobility in a joint due to disease, an injury, or a surgical procedure.
Inflammation of a bursa.	An inflammatory condition of one or more joints.
Abnormal softening of the cartilage.	Stiffening of a joint or joining of spinal vertebrae by surgical means.
The surgical repair of cartilage.	X-ray examination of a joint after the injection of a contrast medium.
A surgical incision or opening into the skull.	The surgical loosening of an ankylosed joint.
A benign growth on the surface of a bone.	The surgical replacement of a joint.
An abnormal increase in the outward curvature of the thoracic spine as viewed from the side.	Stiffness of the joints, especially in the aged.

Lordosis (lor-**DOH**-sis)	**Osteomyelitis** (**oss**-tee-oh-**my**-eh-**LYE**-tis)
Myeloma (**my**-eh-**LOH**-mah)	**Osteoporosis** (**oss**-tee-oh-poh-**ROH**-sis)
Ostealgia (**oss**-tee-**AL**-jee-ah)	**Osteorrhaphy** (**oss**-tee-**OR**-ah-fee)
Osteitis (**oss**-tee-**EYE**-tis)	**Periosteotomy** (**per**-ee-**oss**-tee-**OT**-oh-me)
Osteitis deformans (**oss**-tee-**EYE**-tis dee-**FOR**-manz)	**Periostitis** (**per**-ee-oss-**TYE**-tis)
Osteoclasis (**oss**-tee-**OCK**-lah-sis)	**Scoliosis** (**skoh**-lee-**OH**-sis)
Osteomalacia (**oss**-tee-oh-mah-**LAY**-she-ah)	**Spondylosis** (**spon**-dih-**LOH**-sis)

Activity Cards

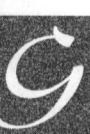

Inflammation of the bone and bone marrow.	An abnormal increase in the forward curvature of the lower or lumbar spine.
A marked loss of bone density and an increase in bone porosity frequently associated with aging.	A tumor composed of cells derived from blood forming tissues of the bone marrow.
The suturing or wiring together of bones.	Any pain linked to an abnormal condition within a bone.
An incision through the periosteum.	Inflammation of bone.
Inflammation of the periosteum.	A disease of unknown cause characterized by extensive bone destruction followed by abnormal bone repair.
An abnormal lateral curvature of the spine.	The surgical fracture of a bone to correct a deformity.
Any degenerative condition of the vertebrae.	Abnormal softening of bones due to disease.

THE MUSCULAR SYSTEM ACTIVITY CARDS

Ataxia (ah-**TACK**-see-ah)	**Fascioplasty** (**fash**-ee-oh-**PLAS**-tee)
Atrophy (**AT**-roh-fee)	**Fasciorrhaphy** (**fash**-ee-**OR**-ah-fee)
Bradykinesia (**brad**-ee-kih-**NEE**-zee-ah)	**Hemiplegia** (**hem**-ee-**PLEE**-jee-ah)
Contracture (kon-**TRACK**-chur)	**Hyperkinesia** (**high**-per-kye-**NEE**-zee-ah)
Dyskinesia (**dis**-kih-**NEE**-zee-ah)	**Hypertonia** (**high**-per-**TOH**-nee-ah)
Dystaxia (dis-**TACK**-see-ah)	**Hypokinesia** (**high**-poh-kye-**NEE**-zee-ah)
Fasciectomy (**fas**-ee-**ECK**-toh-me)	**Hypotonia** (**high**-poh-**TOH**-nee-ah)

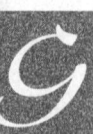

The surgical repair of a fascia.	An inability to coordinate the muscles in the execution of voluntary movement.
The suturing of lacerated fascia.	Weakness and wasting away caused by disuse of the muscle over a long period of time.
The total paralysis of one side of the body.	Extreme slowness in movement.
Abnormally increased motor function or activity.	An abnormal shortening of muscle tissues making the muscle resistant to stretching.
A condition of excessive tone of the skeletal muscles with increased resistance of muscle to passive stretching.	Distortion or impairment of voluntary movement, as in tic, spasm, or myoclonus.
Abnormally decreased motor function or activity.	Difficulty in controlling voluntary movement.
A condition of diminished tone of the skeletal muscles with decreased resistance of muscle to passive stretching.	The surgical removal of fascia.

Myalgia (my-**AL**-jee-ah)	**Myosclerosis** (**my**-oh-skleh-**ROH**-sis)
Myocele (**MY**-oh-seel)	**Myotonia** (**my**-oh-**TOH**-nee-ah)
Myoclonus (**my**-oh-**KLOH**-nus)	**Paraplegia** (**par**-ah-**PLEE**-jee-ah)
Myomalacia (**my**-oh-mah-**LAY**-she-ah)	**Quadriplegia** (**kwad**-rih-**PLEE**-jee-ah)
Myonecrosis (**my**-oh-neh-**KROH**-sis)	**Singultus** (sing-**GUL**-tus)
Myorrhaphy (my-**OR**-ah-fee)	**Tenodesis** (ten-**ODD**-eh-sis)
Myorrhexis (**my**-oh-**RECK**-sis)	**Tenolysis** (ten-**OL**-ih-sis)

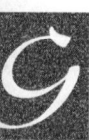

Abnormal hardening of muscle tissue.	Muscle tenderness or pain.
The delayed relaxation of a muscle after a strong contraction.	The protrusion of a muscle through its ruptured sheath or fascia.
The paralysis of both legs and the lower part of the body.	A spasm or twitching of a muscle or group of muscles.
The paralysis of all four extremities.	Abnormal softening of muscle tissue.
Also known as hiccups.	The death of individual muscle fibers.
To suture the end of a tendon or bone.	To suture a muscle wound.
To free a tendon from adhesions.	The rupture of a muscle.

THE CARDIOVASCULAR SYSTEM ACTIVITY CARDS

Aneurysm (**AN**-you-rizm)	**Atherosclerosis** (**ath**-er-**oh**-skleh-**ROH**-sis)
Angina pectoris (an-**JIGH**-nah **PECK**-toh-riss)	**Bradycardia** (**brad**-ee-**KAR**-dee-ah)
Angiography (**an**-jee-**OG**-rah-fee)	**Carditis** (kar-**DYE**-tis)
Angionecrosis (**an**-jee-oh-neh-**KROH**-sis)	**Cardiocentesis** (**kar**-dee-oh-sen-**TEE**-sis)
Arteriectomy (**ar**-teh-ree-**ECK**-toh-me)	**Cardiorrhexis** (**kar**-dee-oh-**RECK**-sis)
Arteriosclerosis (ar-**tee**-ree-oh-skleh-**ROH**-sis)	**Defibrillation** (dee-**fib**-rih-**LAY**-shun)
Arteritis (ar-teh-**RYE**-tis)	**Dyscrasia** (dis-**KRAY**-zee-ah)

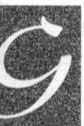

Hardening and narrowing of the arteries due to a buildup of cholesterol plaques.	A localized balloon-like enlargement of an artery.
An abnormally slow heartbeat.	Spasmodic, choking, or suffocating pain that is usually due to interference with the supply of oxygen to the myocardium.
Inflammation of the heart.	A radiographic study of blood vessels after the injection of a radiopaque material.
The puncture of a chamber of the heart for diagnosis or therapy.	The tissue death of the walls of blood vessels.
Rupture of the heart.	The surgical removal of part of an artery.
The use of electrical shock to restore the heart's normal rhythm.	Hardening of the arteries that reduces the flow of blood through these vessels.
Any abnormal or pathologic condition of the blood.	Inflammation of an artery.

Electrocardiography (ee-**leck**-troh-kar-dee-**OG**-rah-fee)	**Mitral stenosis** (**MY**-tral steh-**NO**-sis)
Endarterectomy (**end**-ar-ter-**ECK**-toh-me)	**Myocardial infarction** (**my**-oh-**KAR**-dee-al in-**FARK**-shun)
Endocarditis (**en**-doh-kar-**DYE**-tis)	**Phlebitis** (fleh-**BYE**-tis)
Hemangioma (heh-**man**-jee-**OH**-mah)	**Tachycardia** (**tack**-ee-**KAR**-dee-ah)
Hemostasis (**he**-moh-**STAY**-sis)	**Thrombophlebitis** (**throm**-boh-fleh-**BYE**-tis)
Leukemia (loo-**KEE**-me-ah)	**Valvuloplasty** (**VAL**-view-loh-**plas**-tee)
Leukopenia (**loo**-koh-**PEE**-nee-ah)	**Varicose veins** (**VAR**-ih-kohs **VAYNS**)

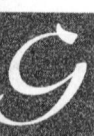

Abnormal narrowing of the opening of the mitral valve.	The process of recording the electrical activity of the myocardium.
Damage to the myocardium that impairs the heart's ability to pump blood through the body.	The surgical removal of plaque from clogged arteries.
Inflammation of a vein.	Inflammation of the inner layer of the heart.
An abnormally fast heartbeat.	A benign tumor made up of newly formed blood vessels.
Inflammation of a vein with a thrombus.	To control bleeding.
The surgical repair of a heart valve.	A malignancy characterized by a progressive increase of abnormal leukocytes.
Abnormally swollen veins usually occurring in the legs.	An abnormal decrease in the number of one or all kinds of white blood cells.

THE IMMUNE SYSTEM AND ONCOLOGY ACTIVITY CARDS

Allergen (AL-er-jen)	**Metastasize** (meh-TAS-tah-sighz)
Antigen (AN-tih-jen)	**Myeloma** (my-eh-LOH-mah)
Autoimmune (aw-toh-ih-MYOUN)	**Myosarcoma** (my-oh-sahr-KOH-mah)
Carcinoma (kar-sih-NO-mah)	**Neuroblastoma** (new-roh-blas-TOH-mah)
Immunodeficiency (im-you-no-deh-FISH-en-see)	**Opportunistic** (op-ur-too-NIHS-tick)
Immunosuppressant (im-you-no-soo-PRES-ant)	**Osteosarcoma** (oss-tee-oh-sar-KOH-mah)
Metastasis (meh-TAS-tah-sis)	**Sarcoma** (sar-KOH-mah)

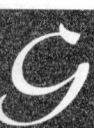

To pass into or invade by the process of metastasis.	A substance capable of inducing an allergic response.
A malignant tumor composed of blood forming tissues of the bone marrow.	Any substance such as a virus, bacterium, or toxin that the body regards as foreign.
A malignant tumor derived from muscle tissue.	A disorder in which the immune system attacks the body's own tissues.
A sarcoma of nervous system origin.	A malignant new growth of epithelial cells that tend to invade surrounding tissues and give rise to metastases.
A pathogen that is able to cause illness because the host's resistance has been decreased by a different disorder.	A disorder in which the immune response is inadequate and resistance to infection is decreased.
A malignant tumor usually involving the upper shaft of long bones, the pelvis, or knee.	A drug that prevents or reduces the body's normal reactions to invasion by disease or foreign tissues.
A malignant neoplasm of the soft tissues arising from supportive and connective tissue.	A pathogenic growth that is distant from the primary disease site.

THE RESPIRATORY SYSTEM ACTIVITY CARDS

Aphonia (ah-**FOH**-nee-ah)	**Dysphonia** (dis-**FOH**-nee-ah)
Apnea (ap-**NEE**-ah)	**Dyspnea** (**DISP**-nee-ah)
Asphyxiation (ass-**fick**-see-**AY**-shun)	**Emphysema** (**em**-fih-**SEE**-mah)
Bronchoplegia (**brong**-koh-**PLEE**-jee-ah)	**Empyema** (**em**-pye-**EE**-mah)
Bronchorrhagia (**brong**-koh-**RAY**-jee-ah)	**Epistaxis** (**ep**-ih-**STACK**-sis)
Bronchorrhea (**brong**-koh-**REE**-ah)	**Hemothorax** (**he**-moh-**THOH**-racks)
Cyanosis (**sigh**-ah-**NO**-sis)	**Hyperventilation** (**high**-per-**ven**-tih-**LAY**-shun)

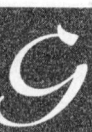

Any voice impairment including hoarseness, weakness, or loss of voice.	Loss of the ability to produce normal speech sounds.
Difficult or labored breathing.	Absence of spontaneous respiration.
Progressive loss of lung function caused by the enlargement of the alveoli.	Any interruption of breathing that may result in the loss of consciousness or death.
An accumulation of pus in the pleural cavity or other body cavities.	Paralysis of the walls of the bronchi.
Bleeding from the nose usually caused by an injury. Also known as a nosebleed.	Bleeding from the bronchi.
An accumulation of blood in the pleural cavity.	Excessive discharge of mucus from the bronchi.
Abnormally rapid deep breathing.	Blue discoloration of the skin caused by a lack of adequate oxygen.

Laryngectomy (lar-in-JECK-toh-me)	**Pneumorrhagia** (new-moh-RAY-jee-ah)
Laryngoplegia (lar-ing-goh-PLEE-jee-ah)	**Pneumothorax** (new-moh-THOR-racks)
Laryngorrhagia (lar-ing-goh-RAY-jee-ah)	**Tracheoplasty** (TRAY-kee-oh-plas-tee)
Laryngospasm (lah-RING-goh-spazm)	**Tracheorrhagia** (tray-kee-oh-RAY-jee-ah)
Pharyngorrhagia (far-ing-goh-RAY-jee-ah)	**Tracheorrhaphy** (tray-kee-OR-ah-fee)
Pharyngorrhea (far-ing-goh-REE-ah)	**Tracheostomy** (tray-kee-OS-toh-me)
Pleurisy (PLOOR-ih-see)	**Tracheotomy** (tray-kee-OT-oh-me)

Activity Cards

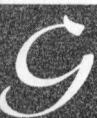

Bleeding from the lungs.	Surgical removal of the larynx.
An accumulation of air or gas in the pleural space causing the lung to collapse.	Paralysis of the larynx.
Surgical repair of the trachea.	Bleeding from the larynx.
Bleeding from the trachea.	A sudden spasmodic closure of the larynx.
Suturing of the trachea.	Bleeding from the pharynx.
Surgical creation of an artifical opening into the trachea.	Discharge of mucus from the pharynx.
A surgical incision into the trachea to gain access to the airway below a blockage.	Inflammation of the visceral and parietal pleura in the thoracic cavity.

THE DIGESTIVE SYSTEM ACTIVITY CARDS

Borborygmus (**bor**-boh-**RIG**-mus)	**Diverticulitis** (**dye**-ver-tick-you-**LYE**-tis)
Cholecystalgia (**koh**-lee-sis-**TAL**-jee-ah)	**Enteritis** (**en**-ter-**EYE**-tis)
Cholecystitis (**koh**-lee-sis-**TYE**-tis)	**Esophageal reflux** (eh-**sof**-ah-**JEE**-al **REE**-flucks)
Cholelithiasis (**koh**-lee-lih-**THIGH**-ah-sis)	**Esophageal varices** (eh-**sof**-ah-**JEE**-al **VAYR**-ih-seez)
Cirrhosis (sir-**ROH**-sis)	**Gastropexy** (**GAS**-troh-**peck**-see)
Colitis (koh-**LYE**-tis)	**Gastrorrhea** (**gas**-troh-**REE**-ah)
Colostomy (koh-**LAHS**-toh-me)	**Gastrorrhexis** (**gas**-troh-**RECK**-sis)

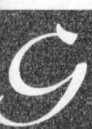

Inflammation of one or more diverticulum.	Rumbling noise caused by the movement of gas in the intestine.
Inflammation of the small intestine.	Pain in the gallbladder.
The return of stomach contents into the esophagus.	Inflammation of the gallbladder.
Enlarged and swollen veins at the lower end of the esophagus.	The presence of gallstones in the gallbladder or bile ducts.
Surgical fixation of the stomach in place to prevent displacement.	A progressive degenerative disease of the liver characterized by disturbance of structure and function of the liver.
The excessive flow of gastric secretions.	Inflammation of the colon.
Rupture of the stomach.	Surgical creation of an opening between the colon and the body surface.

Gastrostomy (gas-**TROS**-toh-me)	**Hyperemesis** (**high**-per-**EM**-eh-sis)
Hematemesis (**hem**-ah-**TEM**-eh-sis)	**Ileectomy** (**ill**-ee-**ECK**-toh-me)
Hepatitis (**hep**-ah-**TYE**-tis)	**Intussusception** (**in**-tus-sus-**SEP**-shun)
Hepatomegaly (**hep**-ah-toh-**MEG**-ah-lee)	**Jaundice** (**JAWN**-dis)
Hepatorrhagia (**hep**-ah-toh-**RAY**-jee-ah)	**Proctopexy** (**PROCK**-toh-**peck**-see)
Hepatorrhea (**hep**-ah-toh-**REE**-ah)	**Pyrosis** (pye-**ROH**-sis)
Hiatal hernia (high-**AY**-tal **HER**-nee-ah)	**Volvulus** (**VOL**-view-lus)

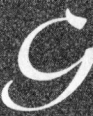

Activity Cards

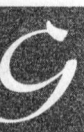

Excessive vomiting.	Surgical creation of an artificial opening into the stomach.
Surgical removal of the ileum.	Vomiting of blood.
Telescoping of one part of the intestine into the opening of an immediately adjacent part.	Inflammation of the liver usually caused by a virus but sometimes from toxic substances.
A yellow discoloration of the skin and other tissues caused by greater than normal amounts of bilirubin in the blood.	An abnormal enlargement of the liver.
Surgical fixation of the rectum to some adjacent tissue or organ.	Bleeding from the liver.
Discomfort due to the regurgitation of stomach acid upward along the esophagus. Also known as heartburn.	Excessive flow of bile from the liver.
Twisting of the intestine upon itself that causes an obstruction.	A protrusion of part of the stomach through the esophageal opening in the diaphragm.

THE URINARY SYSTEM ACTIVITY CARDS

Anuria (ah-**NEW**-ree-ah)	**Diuresis** (**dye**-you-**REE**-sis)
Cystectomy (sis-**TECK**-toh-me)	**Dysuria** (dis-**YOU**-ree-ah)
Cystitis (sis-**TYE**-tis)	**Enuresis** (**en**-you-**REE**-sis)
Cystocele (**SIS**-toh-seel)	**Hydroureter** (**high**-droh-you-**REE**-ter)
Cystopexy (**sis**-toh-**peck**-see)	**Lithotripsy** (**LITH**-oh-**trip**-see)
Cystorrhagia (**sis**-toh-**RAY**-jee-ah)	**Nephrectasis** (neh-**FRECK**-tah-sis)
Dialysis (dye-**AL**-ih-sis)	**Nephrectomy** (neh-**FRECK**-toh-me)

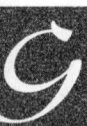

Increased excretion of urine.	Complete suppression of urine formation by the kidneys.
Difficult or painful urination.	Surgical removal of all or part of the urinary bladder.
Involuntary discharge of urine during sleep.	Inflammation of the bladder.
Distention of the ureter with urine, due to blockage from any cause.	A hernia of the bladder through the vaginal wall.
The destruction of a kidney stone with the use of ultrasonic waves traveling through water.	Surgical fixation of the bladder to the abdominal wall.
Distention of a kidney.	Bleeding from the bladder.
Surgical removal of a kidney.	A procedure to remove waste products from the blood of patients whose kidneys no longer function.

Nephrolithiasis (**nef**-row-lih-**THIGH**-ah-sis)	**Pyelitis** (**pye**-eh-**LYE**-tis)
Nephromalacia (**nef**-row-mah-**LAY**-she-ah)	**Pyelotomy** (**pye**-eh-**LOT**-oh-me)
Nephroptosis (**nef**-rop-**TOH**-sis)	**Ureterectasis** (you-**ree**-ter-**ECK**-tah-sis)
Nephropyosis (**nef**-row-pye-**OH**-sis)	**Ureterolith** (you-**REE**-ter-oh-**lith**)
Nocturia (nock-**TOO**-ree-ah)	**Ureterorrhaphy** (**you**-ree-ter-**OR**-ah-fee)
Oliguria (**ol**-ih-**GOO**-ree-ah)	**Urethropexy** (you-**REE**-throh-**peck**-see)
Polyuria (**pol**-ee-**YOU**-ree-ah)	**Urethrorrhea** (you-**ree**-throh-**REE**-ah)

Activity Cards

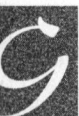

Inflammation of the renal pelvis.	A disorder characterized by the presence of stones in the kidney.
A surgical incision into the renal pelvis.	Abnormal softening of the kidney.
Distention of a ureter.	Prolapse of the kidney.
A stone lodged in a ureter.	Suppuration of the kidney.
To suture a ureter.	Excessive urination during the night.
Surgical fixation of the urethra usually for the correction of urinary stress incontinence.	Scanty urination.
An abnormal discharge from the urethra.	Excessive urination.

THE NERVOUS SYSTEM ACTIVITY CARDS

Alzheimer's (**ALTZ**-high-merz)	**Encephalocele** (en-**SEF**-ah-loh-**seel**)
Aphasia (ah-**FAY**-zee-ah)	**Encephalography** (en-**sef**-ah-**LOG**-rah-fee)
Causalgia (kaw-**ZAL**-jee-ah)	**Epilepsy** (**EP**-ih-**lep**-see)
Cephalalgia (**sef**-ah-**LAL**-jee-ah)	**Hydrocephalus** (high-droh-**SEF**-ah-lus)
Dysphasia (dis-**FAY**-zee-ah)	**Hyperesthesia** (**high**-per-es-**THEE**-zee-ah)
Electroencephalography (ee-**leck**-troh-en-**sef**-ah-**LOG**-rah-fee)	**Meningitis** (**men**-in-**JIGH**-tis)
Encephalitis (**en**-sef-ah-**LYE**-tis)	**Meningocele** (meh-**NING**-goh-**seel**)

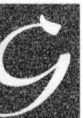

A congenital gap in the skull with herniation of brain substance.	A group of disorders associated with degenerative changes in the brain structure.
A radiographic study demonstrating the intracranial fluid-containing spaces of the brain.	Loss of the ability to speak, write, or comprehend the written or spoken word.
A group of neurologic disorders characterized by recurrent episodes of seizures.	An intense burning pain following an injury to a sensory nerve.
An abnormally increased amount of cerebrospinal fluid within the brain.	Headache or pain in the head.
A condition of excessive sensitivity to stimuli.	An impairment of speech due to a brain lesion.
Inflammation of the meninges of the brain or spinal cord.	The process of recording brain-wave activity.
Protrusion of the membranes of the brain or spinal cord through a defect in the skull or spinal column.	Inflammation of the brain.

Migraine (**MY**-grayn)	**Neurorrhaphy** (new-**ROR**-ah-fee)
Myelitis (**my**-eh-**LYE**-tis)	**Paresthesia** (**par**-es-**THEE**-zee-ah)
Narcolepsy (**NAR**-koh-**lep**-see)	**Poliomyelitis** (**poh**-lee-oh-**my**-eh-**LYE**-tis)
Neuralgia (new-**RAL**-jee-ah)	**Polyneuritis** (**pol**-ee-new-**RYE**-tis)
Neurectomy (new-**RECK**-toh-me)	**Sciatica** (sigh-**AT**-ih-kah)
Neuritis (new-**RYE**-tis)	**Somnambulism** (som-**NAM**-byou-lizm)
Neuroplasty (**NEW**-roh-**plas**-tee)	**Syncope** (**SIN**-koh-pee)

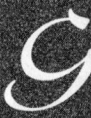

Activity Cards

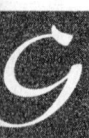

To suture the ends of a severed nerve.	A syndrome characterized by sudden, severe, sharp headache usually present only on one side.
An abnormal sensation, such as burning, tingling, or numbness, for no apparent reason.	Inflammation of the spinal cord. Also inflammation of bone marrow.
A viral infection of the gray matter of the spinal cord that may result in paralysis.	A syndrome characterized by recurrent uncontrollable seizures of drowsiness and sleep.
Inflammation affecting many nerves.	Pain in a nerve or nerves.
Inflammation of the sciatic nerve that may result in pain along the course of the nerve through the thigh and leg.	Surgical removal of a nerve.
The condition of walking without awakening. Also known as sleepwalking.	Inflammation of a nerve or nerves.
The brief loss of consciousness caused by transient cerebral hypoxia. Also known as fainting.	Surgical repair of a nerve or nerves.

THE EYES AND EARS ACTIVITY CARDS

Cataract (**KAT**-ah-rakt)	**Otorrhea** (**oh**-toh-**REE**-ah)
Conjunctivitis (kon-**junk**-tih-**VYE**-tis)	**Phacoemulsification** (**fay**-koh-ee-**mul**-sih-fih-**KAY**-shun)
Glaucoma (glaw-**KOH**-mah)	**Presbycusis** (**pres**-beh-**KOO**-sis)
Macular degeneration (**MACK**-you-lar)	**Presbyopia** (**pres**-bee-**OH**-pee-ah)
Otitis (oh-**TYE**-tis)	**Retinopathy** (**ret**-ih-**NOP**-ah-thee)
Otomycosis (**oh**-toh-my-**KOH**-sis)	**Vertigo** (**VER**-tih-go)
Otopyorrhea (**oh**-toh-**pye**-oh-**REE**-ah)	**Xerophthalmia** (**zeer**-ahf-**THAL**-me-ah)

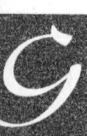

A discharge from the ear.	Cloudiness or the loss of transparency of the lens of the eye.
The use of ultrasonic vibration to shatter and break up a cataract making it easier to remove.	Inflammation of the conjunctiva. Also known as pinkeye.
Progressive hearing loss occurring in old age.	A group of diseases characterized by increased intraocular pressure resulting in damage to the optic nerve and retinal nerve fibers.
Lessening of the accommodation of the lens occurring normally with aging.	A condition in which central vision is lost and peripheral vision may remain.
Any disease of the retina.	Any inflammation of the ear.
A sense of whirling, dizziness and the loss of balance.	A fungus infection of the external auditory canal.
Drying of eye surfaces characterized by the loss of luster of the conjunctiva and cornea.	The flow of pus from the ear.

THE INTEGUMENTARY SYSTEM ACTIVITY CARDS

Actinic keratosis (ack-**TIN**-ick **kerr**-ah-**TOH**-sis)	**Decubitus ulcer** (dee-**KYOU**-bih-tus **UL**-ser)
Alopecia (**al**-oh-**PEE**-shee-ah)	**Dermatomycosis** (**der**-mah-toh-my-**KOH**-sis)
Anhidrosis (**an**-high-**DROH**-sis)	**Ecchymosis** (**eck**-ih-**MOH**-sis)
Blepharoplasty (**BLEF**-ah-roh-**plas**-tee)	**Gangrene** (**GANG**-green)
Bulla (**BULL**-ah)	**Hirsutism** (**HER**-soot-izm)
Cicatrix (sick-**AY**-tricks)	**Hyperhidrosis** (**high**-per-high-**DROH**-sis)
Debridement (day-breed-**MON**)	**Impetigo** (**im**-peh-**TYE**-go)

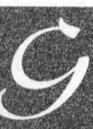

An ulcerated area resulting from prolonged pressure on a body part. Also known as a bedsore.	A precancerous skin lesion caused by excessive exposure to the sun.
A superficial fungal infection of the skin.	A partial or complete lack of hair.
A purplish patch caused by bleeding into the skin. Also known as a bruise.	Condition of lacking or being without sweat.
Tissue death usually associated with a loss of circulation followed by bacterial invasion and putrefaction.	Surgical reduction of the upper and lower eyelids.
Abnormal hairiness.	A large vesicle or blister.
Condition of excessive sweating.	A "normal" scar left by a healed wound.
A contagious superficial pyoderma caused by staphylococci and streptococci.	Removal of dirt, foreign objects, damaged tissue, and cellular debris from a wound.

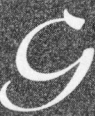

Keloid (**KEE**-loid)	**Purpura** (**PUR**-pew-rah)
Keratosis (**kerr**-ah-**TOH**-sis)	**Rhinophyma** (**rye**-no-**FIGH**-muh)
Lipoma (lih-**POH**-mah)	**Rhinoplasty** (**RYE**-no-**plas**-tee)
Melanosis (**mel**-ah-**NO**-sis)	**Rhytidectomy** (**rit**-ih-**DECK**-toh-me)
Onychomycosis (**on**-ih-koh-my-**KOH**-sis)	**Seborrhea** (**seb**-oh-**REE**-ah)
Plication (plih-**KAY**-shun)	**Urticaria** (**ur**-tih-**KAY**-ree-ah)
Pruritus (proo-**RYE**-tus)	**Xeroderma** (zee-roh-**DER**-mah)

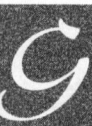

Activity Cards

A condition characterized by hemorrhage into the skin that causes spontaneous bruising.	An abnormally raised or thickened scar.
An overgrowth of skin and oil glands of the nose.	Any benign skin condition in which there is overgrowth and thickening of the epidermis.
Surgery to change the shape or size of the nose.	A benign tumor made up of mature fat cells.
Surgical removal of excess skin for the elimination of wrinkles.	Any condition of unusual deposits of black pigment in different parts of the body.
Any of several common skin conditions in which there is an over production of sebum.	A fungus infection of the nail.
Localized areas of swelling accompanied by itching that is associated with an allergic reaction.	A surgical procedure of taking tucks in a structure to shorten it.
Excessively dry skin.	Itching.

THE ENDOCRINE SYSTEM ACTIVITY CARDS

Acromegaly (**ack**-roh-**MEG**-ah-lee)	**Hypogonadism** (**high**-poh-**GO**-nad-izm)
Cretinism (**CREE**-tin-izm)	**Hypothyroidism** (**high**-poh-**THIGH**-roid-izm)
Hypercrinism (**high**-per-**KRY**-nism)	**Pituitarism** (pih-**TOO**-ih-tar-izm)
Hypergonadism (**high**-per-**GO**-nad-izm)	**Thymitis** (thigh-**MY**-tis)
Hyperinsulinism (**high**-per-**IN**-suh-lin-izm)	**Thymoma** (thigh-**MOH**-mah)
Hyperpituitarism (**high**-per-pih-**TOO**-ih-tah-rizm)	**Thyromegaly** (**thigh**-roh-**MEG**-ah-lee)
Hypocrinism (**high**-poh-**KRY**-nism)	**Thyrotoxicosis** (**thy**-roh-**tock**-sih-**KOH**-sis)

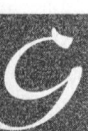

The condition of deficient secretion of hormones by the sex glands.	Enlargement of the extremities (hands and feet) caused by excessive secretion of the growth hormone after puberty.
A deficiency of thyroid secretion.	Arrested physical and mental development due to a congenital lack of thyroid secretion.
Any disorder of pituitary function.	A condition caused by excessive secretion of any gland, especially an endocrine gland.
Inflammation of the thymus gland.	The condition of excessive secretion of hormones by the sex glands.
A benign tumor derived from the tissue of the thymus.	Excessive insulin in the bloodstream that may cause insulin shock.
An abnormal enlargement of the thyroid gland causing a swelling in the front part of the neck.	A condition due to excessive secretion of the pituitary gland.
A life-threatening condition resulting from the presence of excessive quantities of the thyroid hormones.	A condition caused by deficient secretion of any gland, especially an endocrine gland.

THE MALE REPRODUCTIVE SYSTEM ACTIVITY CARDS

Anorchism (an-**OR**-kizm)	**Impotence** (**IM**-poh-tens)
Azoospermia (ay-**zoh**-oh-**SPER**-me-ah)	**Oligospermia** (**ol**-ih-goh-**SPER**-me-ah)
Benign prostatic hypertrophy	**Orchidectomy** (**or**-kih-**DECK**-toh-me)
Circumcision (**ser**-kum-**SIZH**-un)	**Prostatorrhea** (**pros**-tah-toh-**REE**-ah)
Cryptorchidism (krip-**TOR**-kih-dizm)	**Testitis** (test-**TYE**-tis)
Epididymitis (**ep**-ih-did-ih-**MY**-tis)	**Transurethral prostatectomy** (**trans**-you-**REE**-thral **pros**-tah-**TECK**-toh-me)
Hydrocele (**HIGH**-droh-seel)	**Vasectomy** (vah-**SECK**-toh-me)

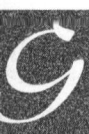

Inability of the male to achieve or maintain a penile erection.	Congenital absence of one or both testicles.
A deficient amount of sperm in the semen.	Absence of sperm in the semen.
Surgical removal of a testis.	An overgrowth of the glandular tissue of the prostate.
An abnormal flow of prostatic fluid discharged through the urethra.	Surgical removal of the foreskin of the penis.
Inflammation of a testis.	A developmental defect in which one testis fails to descend into the scrotum.
Surgical removal of all or part of the prostate through the urethra.	Inflammation of the epididymis.
Male sterilization procedure in which a portion of the vas or ductus deferens is surgically removed.	A hernia or fluid in the testes or the tubes leading from the testes.

PREGNANCY AND CHILDBIRTH ACTIVITY CARDS

Abruptio placentae (ab-**RUP**-she-oh plah-**SEN**-tee)	**Nulligravida** (**null**-ih-**GRAV**-ih-dah)
Amniocentesis (**am**-nee-oh-sen-**TEE**-sis)	**Nullipara** (nuh-**LIP**-ah-rah)
Eclampsia (eh-**KLAMP**-see-ah)	**Parturition** (**par**-tyou-**RISH**-un)
Episiorrhaphy (eh-**piz**-ee-**OR**-ah-fee)	**Placenta previa** (plah-**SEN**-tah **PREE**-vee-ah)
Episiotomy (eh-**piz**-ee-**OT**-oh-me)	**Preeclampsia** (**pree**-ee-**KLAMP**-see-ah)
Meconium (meh-**KOH**-nee-um)	**Primigravida** (**pre**-mih-**GRAV**-ih-dah)
Multiparous (mul-**TIP**-ah-rus)	**Primipara** (prye-**MIP**-ah-rah)

Activity Cards

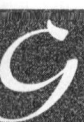

A woman who has never been pregnant.	An abnormal condition in which the placenta separates from the uterine wall prematurely before the birth of the fetus.
A woman who has never borne a viable child.	A diagnostic test to evaluate fetal health and diagnose certain congenital disorders.
Childbirth; labor; the act of giving birth to an offspring.	More serious form of preeclampsia, characterized by convulsions and sometimes coma.
The abnormal implantation of the placenta in the lower portion of the uterus.	Sutured repair of an episiotomy.
A complication of pregnancy characterized by hypertension, edema, and proteinuria.	A surgical incision of the perineum and vagina to facilitate delivery and prevent laceration of the tissues.
A woman during her first pregnancy.	Material that collects in the intestine of a fetus and forms the first stools of a newborn.
A woman who has borne one child.	A woman who has given birth two or more times.

THE FEMALE REPRODUCTIVE SYSTEM ACTIVITY CARDS

Amenorrhea (ah-**men**-oh-**REE**-ah)	**Endometriosis** (**en**-doh-**me**-tree-**OH**-sis)
Cervicectomy (**ser**-vih-**SECK**-toh-me)	**Hypomenorrhea** (**high**-poh-men-oh-**REE**-ah)
Colpitis (kol-**PYE**-tis)	**Hysterectomy** (**hiss**-teh-**RECK**-toh-me)
Colpopexy (**KOL**-poh-**peck**-see)	**Hysteropexy** (**HISS**-ter-oh-**peck**-see)
Colporrhaphy (kol-**POR**-ah-fee)	**Hysterorrhaphy** (**hiss**-ter-**OR**-ah-fee)
Conization (**kon**-ih-**ZAY**-shun)	**Leukorrhea** (**loo**-koh-**REE**-ah)
Dysmenorrhea (**dis**-men-oh-**REE**-ah)	**Mastopexy** (**MAS**-toh-**peck**-see)

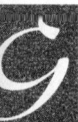

A condition in which endometrial tissue escapes the uterus and becomes implanted outside the uterus on other structures in the pelvic cavity.	Absence of the monthly flow of menstruation.
A small amount of menstrual flow over a shortened duration at the regular period.	Surgical removal of the cervix.
Surgical removal of the uterus.	Inflammation of the vagina.
Surgical fixation of a misplaced or abnormally movable uterus.	Surgical fixation of the vagina to a surrounding structure.
To suture the uterus.	Suturing the vagina.
A profuse white mucous discharge from the uterus and vagina.	Removal of a cone of tissue or the partial removal of the cervix.
Surgery to affix sagging breasts in a more elevated position.	Difficult or painful monthly flow.

Menometrorrhagia (men-oh-met-roh-RAY-jee-ah)	**Oophoroplasty** (oh-OF-oh-plas-tee)
Menorrhagia (men-oh-RAY-jee-ah)	**Ovariorrhexis** (oh-vay-ree-oh-RECK-sis)
Metrorrhea (me-troh-REE-ah)	**Papanicolaou test** (pap-ah-nick-oh-LAY-ooh)
Metrorrhexis (me-troh-RECK-sis)	**Polymenorrhea** (pol-ee-men-oh-REE-ah)
Mittelschmerz (MIT-uhl-schmehrts)	**Pruritus vulvae** (proo-RYE-tus VUL-vee)
Oligomenorrhea (ol-ih-goh-men-oh-REE-ah)	**Vaginitis** (vaj-ih-NIGH-tis)
Oophoritis (oh-of-oh-RYE-tis)	**Vaginocele** (VAJ-ih-no-seel)

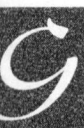

Surgical repair of an ovary.	Excessive uterine bleeding occurring both during the menses and at irregular intervals.
Rupture of an ovary.	Excessive uterine bleeding occurring during the menses.
An exfoliative test for the detection and diagnosis of conditions of the cervix and surrounding tissues.	An abnormal uterine discharge.
Abnormally frequent menstruation.	Rupture of the uterus.
A condition of severe itching of the external female genitalia.	Pain between menstrual periods that usually occurs at the time of ovulation.
Inflammation of the vagina.	A markedly reduced menstrual flow; abnormally infrequent menstruation or relative amenorrhea.
A hernia protruding into the vagina.	Inflammation of an ovary.

EXAMINATION TERMINOLOGY ACTIVITY CARDS

Abdominocentesis (ab-**dom**-ih-no-sen-**TEE**-sis)	**Phlebotomy** (fleh-**BOT**-oh-me)
Auscultation (**aws**-kul-**TAY**-shun)	**Rale** (**RAHL**)
Bruit (**BREW**-ee)	**Rhonchus** (**RONG**-kus)
Ophthalmoscope (ahf-**THAL**-moh-skope)	**Speculum** (**SPECK**-you-lum)
Otoscope (**OH**-toh-skope)	**Sphygmomanometer** (**sfig**-moh-mah-**NOM**-eh-ter)
Palpation (pal-**PAY**-shun)	**Stethoscope** (**STETH**-oh-skope)
Percussion (per-**KUSH**-un)	**Thoracentesis** (**thoh**-rah-sen-**TEE**-sis)

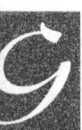

The puncture of a vein for the purpose of drawing blood.	The surgical puncture of the abdominal cavity.
An abnormal rattle or crackle-like respiratory sound heard during inspiration (breathing in).	Listening through a stethoscope for sounds within the body to determine the condition of the lungs, pleura, heart, and abdomen.
The respiratory sound caused by air passing through bronchi that are narrowed. Also known as a **wheeze**.	A sound or murmur heard in auscultation, especially an abnormal one.
An instrument used to enlarge the opening of any canal or cavity to facilitate inspection of its interior.	An instrument used to examine the interior of the eye.
An instrument used to measure blood pressure.	An instrument used to visually examine the external ear canal and tympanic membrane.
An instrument used to listen to blood sounds within the body.	An examination technique in which the examiner's hands are used to feel the texture, size, consistency, and location of certain body parts.
The puncture of the chest wall to obtain fluid for diagnostic purposes, to drain pleural effusions, or to reexpand a collapsed lung.	A diagnostic procedure to determine the density of a body area by the sound produced by tapping the surface with the finger or instrument.

ENDOSCOPIC EXAMINATION ACTIVITY CARDS

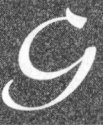

Endoscopy (en-**DOS**-koh-pee)	**Esophagoscopy** (eh-**sof**-ah-**GOS**-koh-pee)
Anoscopy (ah-**NOS**-koh-pee)	**Gastroscope** (**GAS**-troh-skope)
Arthroscopy (ar-**THROS**-koh-pee)	**Hysteroscope** (**HISS**-ter-oh-skope)
Bronchoscopy (brong-**KOS**-koh-pee)	**Laparoscopy** (**lap**-ah-**ROS**-koh-pee)
Colonoscopy (**koh**-lun-**OSS**-koh-pee)	**Laryngoscopy** (**lar**-ing-**GOS**-koh-pee)
Colposcopy (kol-**POS**-koh-pee)	**Sigmoidoscope** (sig-**MOI**-doh-skope)
Cystoscopy (sis-**TOS**-koh-pee)	

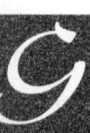

Visual examination or treatment of the esophagus using an esophagoscope.	The visual examination or treatment of the interior of any cavity of the body by means of an endoscope.
An instrument used for the visual examination or treatment of the stomach.	Visual examination or treatment of the anal canal and lower rectum using an anoscope.
Instrument used in direct visual examination of the interior of the uterus.	Visual examination or treatment of the internal structure of a joint using an arthroscope.
The visual examination or treatment of the interior of the abdomen using a laparoscope.	Visual examination or treatment of the bronchi using a bronchoscope.
Visual examination or treatment of the larynx using a laryngoscope.	Visual examination or treatment of the inner surface of the colon, from the rectum to the cecum using a colonoscope.
An instrument used for the visual examination or treatment of the interior of the entire rectum, sigmoid colon, and possibly a portion of the descending colon.	Visual examination or treatment of the tissues of the cervix and vagina using a colposcope.
	Visual examination or treatment of the urinary bladder using a cystoscope.

GENERAL MEDICAL TERMINOLOGY ACTIVITY CARDS

Acronym (**ACK**-roh-nim)	**Eponym** (**EP**-oh-nim)
Amnesia (am-**NEE**-zee-ah)	**Hallucination** (hah-**loo**-sih-**NAY**-shun)
Communicable (kuh-**MEW**-nih-kuh-bul)	**Iatrogenic** (eye-**at**-roh-**JEN**-ick)
Delirium (dee-**LIR**-ee-um)	**Idiopathic** (**id**-ee-oh-**PATH**-ick)
Empathy (**EM**-pah-thee)	**Nosocomial** (**nos**-oh-**KOH**-me-al)
Endemic (en-**DEM**-ick)	**Pandemic** (pan-**DEM**-ick)
Epidemic (**ep**-ih-**DEM**-ick)	**Syndrome** (**SIN**-drome)

Activity Cards

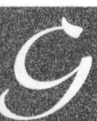

The name of a disease, structure, operation, or procedure, usually derived from the name of the person who discovered or described it first.	A word formed from the initial letter or letters of the major parts of a compound term.
A sense perception that has no basis in external stimulation.	A disturbance in the memory marked by total or partial inability to recall past experiences.
An unfavorable response to medical or surgical treatment, induced by the treatment itself.	Any disease transmitted from one person to another either by direct contact or indirectly by contact with contaminated objects.
An illness without known cause.	A disturbance of consciousness characterized by a change in cognition that developed over a short period of time.
A hospital-acquired infection that was not present on admission that appears 72 hours or more after hospitalization.	The ability to identify with another person's mental and emotional state.
A disease outbreak occurring over a large geographic area, possibly worldwide.	The ongoing presence of a disease within a population, group, or area.
A set of the signs and symptoms that occur together as part of a specific disease process.	A sudden and widespread outbreak of a disease within a population group or area.

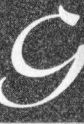

Activity Cards

Activity Cards

SECTION H

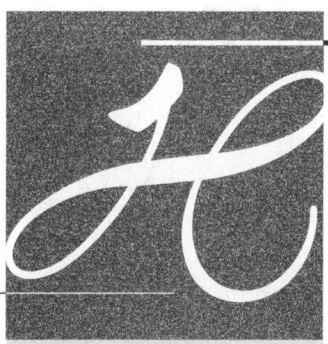

Case Studies

Overview of Case Studies

- **Case 1 History and Physical Examination, Operative Report, and Discharge Summary**
  Body system(s): Digestive system. Follows a patient through the diagnosis and treatment of appendicitis
  Comments: This is an excellent introduction to case studies because it follows one patient through three phases of treatment

- **Case 2 History and Physical Examination**
  Body system(s): Cardiovascular system
  Impression: Possible congestive heart failure

- **Case 3 Radiology Report**
  Body system(s): Respiratory system
  Procedure: Chest x-ray

- **Case 4 Ultrasound Report**
  Body system(s): Urinary system
  Procedure: Prostate ultrasound

- **Case 5 Case Summary**
  Body system(s): Oncology and skeletal system
  Comment: Ongoing treatment for Ewing's sarcoma

- **Case 6 Case Summary**
  Body system(s): Endocrine system (diabetes mellitus), cardiovascular system (congestive heart failure and hypertension), and urinary system (renal failure)
  Comment: This summary shows how one disorder (diabetes mellitus) causes problems with other body systems

- **Case 7 Consultation Report**
  Body system(s): Nervous system and special senses
  Reason for consultation: Eye infection

- **Case 8 Consultation Report**
  Body system(s): Immune system
  Reason for consultation: Allergy

- **Case 9 Consultation Report**
  Body system(s): Nervous system and special senses
  Reason for consultation: Patient's primary complaint was paroxysmal positional vertigo (dizziness)

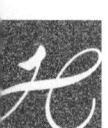

- **Case 10   Consultation Report**
  Body system(s): Cardiovascular system (anemia), immune system (autoimmune disease, i.e. rheumatoid arthritis), skeletal system (rheumatoid arthritis)
  Reason for consultation: Anemia and possible underlying autoimmune process

- **Case 11   Consultation Report**
  Body system(s): Immune system
  Reason for consultation: Ongoing consultation for patient with AIDS

- **Case 12   Consultation Report**
  Body system(s): Nervous system and special senses
  Reason for consultation: Cataract surgery and follow-up care
  Note: This type of report is also referred to as a *courtesy letter*.

- **Case 13   Operative Report**
  Body system(s): Digestive system
  Procedure: Total colonoscopy

- **Case 14   Operative Report**
  Body system(s): Urinary system
  Procedure: Cystoscopy

- **Case 15   Operative Report**
  Body system(s): Skeletal system
  Procedure: Open reduction of a fracture

- **Case 16   Operative Report**
  Body system(s): Reproductive system
  Procedure: Cesarean section

- **Case 17   Operative Report**
  Body system(s): Cardiovascular system
  Procedure: Femoral artery bypass

- **Case 18   Operative Report**
  Body system(s): Oncology and urinary system
  Procedure: Removal of Wilms' tumor of the left kidney

- **Case 19   Operative Report**
  Body system(s): Oncology and reproductive system. Breast cancer
  Procedure: Modified radical mastectomy

- **Case 20   Discharge Summary**
  Body system(s): Digestive system
  Primary discharge diagnosis: Colostomy closure

- **Case 21   Discharge Summary**
  Body system(s): Digestive system
  Primary discharge diagnosis: Sigmoid diverticulitis

- **Case 22   Discharge Summary**
  Body system(s): Skeletal system
  Primary discharge diagnosis: Multiple compression fractures

- **Case 23   Discharge Summary**
  Body system(s): Respiratory system
  Primary discharge diagnosis: Pneumonia

- **Case 24   Discharge Summary**
  Body system(s): Endocrine system (diabetes mellitus and hypothyroidism), and cardiovascular system (cardiac arrhythmia and hyperlipidemia)
  Primary discharge diagnosis: Ventricular tachycardia

CASE 1

HISTORY AND PHYSICAL EXAMINATION

PATIENT NAME: Jonathan Jones　　　　　　　　　　　　MR#: 44579

ATTENDING PHYSICIAN: P. Smith, M.D.　　　　　　　ROOM#: 527-A

CHIEF COMPLAINT: Abdominal pain.

HISTORY OF PRESENT ILLNESS: The patient is a 27-year-old Caucasian male complaining of right lower quadrant abdominal pain, nausea, and vomiting. The initial onset of the pain was about 48 hours prior to presentation, when he became aware of abdominal discomfort. The pain was progressive in nature and began radiating to the back. Late yesterday, the patient drank some Alka-Seltzer and went to bed. He was awakened during the night by the pain and began vomiting. The patient states the pain is constant and has localized to the right lower quadrant. His last bowel movement yesterday afternoon was normal. He does have a history of irritable bowel syndrome. However, he states that this pain is different from the pain he has had in the past.

PAST MEDICAL HISTORY: Irritable bowel syndrome, last exacerbation 6 months ago. The rest of the past medical history is unremarkable.

PAST SURGICAL HISTORY: Tonsillectomy and adenoidectomy in early childhood. Umbilical hernia repair at age 4.

MEDICATIONS: None.

ALLERGIES: No known drug allergies.

SOCIAL HISTORY: The patient is employed as a computer programmer. He is married and has no children. He has smoked a half pack of cigarettes daily for the last five years. He drinks alcohol rarely.

FAMILY HISTORY: Both parents are alive and well. One sister has Down syndrome.

REVIEW OF SYSTEMS: Negative except for complaint of pain in the right lower quadrant.

PHYSICAL EXAMINATION:

GENERAL: The patient is an alert, oriented white male appearing his stated age. He appears to be in moderate distress. Vital signs: blood pressure 132/78. Pulse 68 and regular. Temperature 101.4° Fahrenheit.

CASE 1

HISTORY AND PHYSICAL EXAMINATION (cont.)

HEENT: Normocephalic, nontraumatic. Pupils were equal, round, reactive to light. Ears clear. Throat normal.

NECK: The neck is supple with no carotid bruits.

LUNGS: The lungs are clear to auscultation and percussion.

HEART: Regular rate and rhythm.

ABDOMEN: Bowel sounds are normal. There is rebound tenderness, with maximal discomfort on palpation in the right lower quadrant.

EXTREMITIES: No clubbing, cyanosis, or edema.

LABORATORY DATA: Hemoglobin 14.6, hematocrit 43.6, WBC 13,000. Sodium 138, potassium 3.8, chloride 105, CO_2 24, BUN 10, creatinine 0.9, glucose 102. The urinalysis was negative.

DIAGNOSTIC STUDIES: Flat plate and upright films of the abdomen revealed a localized abnormal gas pattern in the right lower quadrant with no evidence of free air.

IMPRESSION: Appendicitis.

PLAN: The patient will be admitted and an appendectomy will be performed by Dr. Rogers.

Phyllis Smith, M.D.

PS/LM

CASE 1

OPERATIVE REPORT

PATIENT NAME: Jonathan Jones   MR#: 44579

ATTENDING PHYSICIAN: P. Smith, M.D.   ROOM#: 527-A

SURGEON: F. Rogers, M.D.   DATE: 9-2-XX

PREOPERATIVE DIAGNOSIS: Appendicitis.
POSTOPERATIVE DIAGNOSIS: Appendicitis.
ANESTHESIA: General endotracheal.
PROCEDURE: Appendectomy.

INDICATIONS: The patient is a 27-year-old white male with a history of progressively worsening abdominal pain, which localized to the right lower quadrant. The patient later developed nausea and vomiting. Based on the history and physical examination, and initial laboratory and diagnostic studies, it was felt the patient had appendicitis. It was decided to keep him NPO overnight and proceed with surgery in the early morning.

The procedure, its risks, and possible complications were fully explained and the patient signed the appropriate consent forms.

PROCEDURE: The patient was prepared and draped in the usual sterile manner. General endotracheal anesthetic was administered. The abdomen was entered with a Rocky-Davis incision using a #10 blade. Hemostasis was obtained with electrocautery. A muscle-splitting incision was made and carried down to the peritoneum. The peritoneum was grasped with two hemostats and a small incision was made with a #10 scalpel. The cecum was grasped with a Babcock forceps and delivered through the wound. The appendix was grossly inflamed and obviously acute. It was excised and sutured and the base inverted into the stump. The appendix was sent to pathology. On limited exploration of the adjacent areas, there were no abnormal findings. The wound was then thoroughly irrigated. The posterior fascia was then closed with a running suture of #1 Prolene. The anterior fascia was closed in the same manner. The skin was closed with staples. A sterile dressing was applied.

The patient tolerated the procedure well and went to the recovery room in satisfactory condition.

_____

Francine Rogers, M.D.

FR/LM

CASE 1

DISCHARGE SUMMARY

PATIENT NAME: Jonathan Jones   MR#: 44579

ATTENDING PHYSICIAN: P. Smith, M.D.   ROOM#: 527-A

ADMISSION DATE: 9-1-91   DISCHARGE DATE: 9-5-91

DISCHARGE DIAGNOSIS: Appendicitis.
PROCEDURE: Appendectomy.
COMPLICATIONS: None.

HISTORY: The patient is a 27-year-old white male who was admitted complaining of pain localized to the right lower quadrant, associated with nausea, vomiting, and fever. He was admitted through the emergency room after the diagnosis of appendicitis was made and kept NPO.

HOSPITAL COURSE: The morning following admission, the patient was taken to the operating room where Dr. Rogers removed an acute appendix without complications.

Over the next 48 hours, the patient experienced steady improvement, responding well to fluids and oral antibiotics, and progressing rapidly to a normal diet. His temperature returned to normal within 24 hours of the procedure.

LABORATORY DATA: CBC was within normal limits. Flat plate of the abdomen was normal.

DISCHARGE MEDICATIONS: The patient was given a prescription for Tylenol #3 to be taken as needed for pain.

DISPOSITION: The patient is discharged home in good condition, with instructions to return to my office in 1 week for suture removal and follow-up care.

                                                    Phyllis Smith, M.D.

PS/LM

Case 1 Study Questions

1. What three reports make up this case study and why is each important?
2. What does the abbreviation HEENT mean?
3. What surgeries are listed in the patient's past surgical history?
4. The extremities are described as "No clubbing, cyanosis, or edema." What do each of these terms mean?
5. The operative report states that "hemostasis was obtained with electrocautery." What does this mean?

CASE 2

HISTORY AND PHYSICAL EXAMINATION

RE: Carla Mason   DATE: 8-8-XX

REF. PHYS.: Janice Baker, M.D.

I had the pleasure of seeing Mrs. Mason at your request.

HISTORY: She is a 48-year-old black female who states she was doing well until about 1 month ago, when she developed dyspnea on exertion as well as PND and orthopnea. She also complained of peripheral edema over that period of time. The patient gives a history of atypical-type chest discomfort located over the left breast, described as a dull ache. There is no relationship to exertion nor is it relieved by rest. She denies a prior history of coronary artery disease or prior history of myocardial infarction.

Her risk factors are negative for hypertension or diabetes mellitus. She does admit to tobacco use, one and one-half to two packs per day.

FAMILY HISTORY: Her family history is negative for coronary artery disease.

ALLERGIES: None.

MEDICATIONS: Medications include Lanoxin 0.125 mg daily, Slow-K 8 mEq t.i.d., Lasix 40 mg a day.

OPERATIVE HISTORY: She gives a history of cholecystectomy. Carcinoma of the colon was discovered in the early 1980s. She had a total abdominal hysterectomy in 1974, secondary to carcinoma of the uterus. She has had four C-sections. She also gives a history of cysts involving the right kidney.

The patient gives a history of having been on chemotherapy for about 9 months for carcinoma of the colon.

PHYSICAL EXAMINATION:

GENERAL: She is a well-nourished, well-developed, obese black female in no acute distress. Blood pressure was 130/80, pulse was 100 and regular. Her weight was 213 pounds.

HEENT: Head is nontraumatic, normocephalic. Eyes: pupils equal, round and reactive to light, the sclera was clear, the conjunctiva was pink.

NECK: Supple. There is a good carotid upstroke noted bilaterally. The thyroid was noted to be midline. No bruits were appreciated.

CASE 2

HISTORY AND PHYSICAL EXAMINATION (cont.)

CHEST AND LUNGS: Clear to A&P without rales, rhonchi, or wheezes appreciated.

CARDIAC: PMI was found to be normal, S1 and S2 heard, no S3. No murmurs were appreciated.

ABDOMEN: The abdomen revealed multiple scars in the abdomen as well as in the pelvis. Bowel sounds were audible and felt to be normal. I was unable to palpate the liver or spleen.

EXTREMITIES: Negative for cyanosis, clubbing, or edema.

IMPRESSION: The history is compatible with congestive heart failure. However, at this time the patient is not in congestive heart failure. This most likely is secondary to the fact that she is on Lanoxin, Lasix, and Slow-K. Except for smoking, the patient does not have any risk factors. I have proceeded to evaluate her cardiac function by ordering a chest x-ray to evaluate cardiac size, an echocardiogram with Doppler to evaluate left ventricular function, and a stress test with thallium to evaluate for the presence of coronary artery disease.

Thank you very much for allowing me to see this patient. After the studies have been completed, a follow-up letter will be forwarded.

L.E. Bergeron, M.D.

LEB/LM

Case 2 Study Questions

1. The history states that the patient developed dyspnea. What does this mean?
2. What does the abbreviation PND mean?
3. The patient has a history of cholecystectomy. What does this mean?
4. The patient has a history of colon cancer. How was it treated?
5. The physician plans to order an echocardiogram with Doppler. What does this mean?

CASE 3

RADIOLOGY REPORT

PATIENT NAME: Peter Ventura   MR#: 900458

ATTENDING PHYSICIAN: Margaret Majors, M.D.   ROOM: OPD

DATE: 11-12-XX

PROCEDURE: PA and Lateral Chest

INDICATIONS: Weakness, rule out AIDS, *Pneumocystis carinii* pneumonia. The patient has had difficulty breathing and has been losing weight. No old films available for comparison.

FINDINGS: Underlying COPD is noted. The heart size appears normal. The pulmonary vessels appear unremarkable. There is no evidence of pleural effusion.

Extensive interstitial infiltrates are present throughout both lungs. The findings are consistent with diffuse bilateral interstitial pneumonia, probably interstitial fibrosis. The lungs are hyperinflated and there are emphysematous changes in both upper lobes, more prominent on the right.

IMPRESSION: COPD with bullous emphysema. Severe diffuse interstitial lung disease, most likely interstitial fibrosis. *Pneumocystis carinii* pneumonia should be considered in the differential diagnosis.

R. Patchka, M.D.

RP/LM

Case 3 Study Questions

1. What two radiographic views were taken of this patient's chest?
2. What does the abbreviation COPD mean?
3. There was no evidence of pleural effusion. What does this mean?
4. The term "rule out" is used in this report. What does this mean?
5. Extensive interstitial infiltrates are present. What does the term interstitial mean?

CASE 4

ULTRASOUND REPORT

PATIENT NAME: Darnell Wysmith DATE: 9-4-XX

REF. PHYSICIAN: A. Benderman, M.D.

With the patient in the left lateral decubitus position, a digital rectal examination was performed. The prostate was +/- in size, benign in character, soft, symmetrical, and without nodules.

The Proscan ultrasound probe was inserted in the rectum with ease. The prostate was scanned in a transverse fashion. The seminal vesicles appeared normal. As we descended on the base of the prostate, it was obvious that there was a hypoechoic area on the right. It was located in the central zone, possibly involving the peripheral zone, but not in the usual area for carcinoma.

Dimensions of the area were obtained. The diameter was 1.4 cm and 1.2 on another measurement. The area was marked and permanent images obtained. Further examination revealed a calcific density more toward the apex on the right. At the apex, the urethra was prominent and appeared normal. Longitudinal sections were obtained. The apex was intact and the gland was quite small. The entire gland could easily be encompassed in one image. The seminal vesicles in the junction of the seminal vesical and base of the prostate appeared normal without evidence of disease.

Using the Biopty gun, the scanner was set on the hypoechoic area described above. Two biopsies were obtained from this area—one on the right in a random fashion toward the apex and one random biopsy from the left. The dimensions of the prostate were: volume 20.2 ml with a diameter of 4.9 cm. The procedure was concluded.

Sam Metzenbaum, M.D.

SM/LM

Case 4 Study Questions

1. What is the prostate, where is it located, and what is its function?
2. How does an ultrasound examination differ from a radiograph, an MRI, and an endoscopic examination?
3. The report stated that the patient was in a decubitus position. What does this mean?
4. The report states that permanent images were obtained of specific areas. What does this mean?
5. A calcific density was located. What does this mean?

CASE 5

CASE SUMMARY

PATIENT NAME: Vernon Anderson   **MR#:** 0030409

ATTENDING PHYSICIAN: A. Knightly

REASON FOR ADMISSION: Continued treatment of Ewing's sarcoma of the right proximal humerus.

HISTORY OF PRESENT ILLNESS: The patient is a 22-year-old white male with Ewing's sarcoma of the right humerus diagnosed in November 1990, after a pathologic fracture and subsequent biopsy revealed Ewing's sarcoma. The patient was on limited stage disease in work-up and was begun on the experimental arm of the TOG protocol with ifosfamide and etoposide alternating with VAC. A repeat evaluation in January 1991, prior to cycle four, revealed a normal chest CT, CT of the right humerus with increased calcification with healing of the pathologic fracture site. Bone scan was normal. Since then, the patient received cycle 5 without complications. He has received local x-ray therapy to the right humerus, which was recently completed. The patient now presents for cycle 6 of his ifosfamide etoposide with mesna for prevention of hemorrhagic cystitis. The patient is presently without complaints.

MEDICATIONS: Zantac 150 mg p.o. b.i.d.

SOCIAL HISTORY: No smoking or alcohol abuse.

PHYSICAL EXAMINATION: He was a well-developed, well-nourished white gentleman in no acute distress. Temperature 97.6, pulse 76, respiratory rate 16, BP 120/72. The physical exam was significant for alopecia. He had no adenopathy. His lungs were clear. His heart was normal. Abdomen was soft and nontender. The right humerus was without tenderness with full range of motion, pulses 2+. He has some erythema over his right shoulder and proximal humerus area and in the area of his x-ray port was a healing bolus from his XRT. Neurologic revealed he was alert and oriented x3 and nonfocal.

ADMISSION LABORATORY: White count 4.8, hemoglobin 10.3, hematocrit 31.7, platelets 637,000. Chem 1 revealed sodium 140, potassium 4.3, chloride 104, bicarb 26.5, BUN 9, creatinine 1.0, glucose 81. Urinalysis normal. Chest x-ray normal.

HOSPITAL COURSE: The patient was admitted and began cycle 6 and received 5 days of ifosfamide, etoposide with mesna. The patient tolerated his chemotherapy well during the 5 days with minimal nausea and vomiting. His hydration remained good. His urine output remained good and his labs remained within normal limits during his hospital stay. The patient received an MRI and CT scan of his right shoulder and

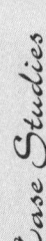

CASE 5

CASE SUMMARY (cont.)

plain films of his right shoulder, which showed continued callus formation with evidence of healing. The MRI and CT scan showed no evidence of change from February 1991, so that there was no evidence of tumor and healing.

DISCHARGE DIAGNOSES:
1. Ewing's sarcoma, right humerus, presently cycle 6 completion of ifosfamide and etoposide.
2. History of pathologic fracture of the right humerus secondary to #1.

PROCEDURES: Bone scan, MRI right shoulder. CT scan right shoulder and humerus.

DISCHARGE MEDICATIONS: Compazine 10 mg p.o. q. 6–8 hours, p.r.n. nausea and vomiting.

DISPOSITION: The patient is discharged to continue his treatment as an outpatient. He will follow-up with Dr. Knightly in the Hematology/Oncology Clinic in 1 week for counts. The patient will also receive an orthopedic evaluation as an outpatient to determine the status of his healing pathologic fracture.

A. Knightly, M.D.

Case 5 Study Questions

1. What is Ewing's sarcoma and what body part is involved in this patient?
2. Why was this patient hospitalized at this time?
3. The physical examination was significant for alopecia. What does this mean?
4. In addition to the chemotherapy, what localized treatment has the patient received for this disease?
5. A bone scan, MRI, and CT scan were performed. How do these diagnostic tests differ?

CASE 6

CASE SUMMARY

PATIENT NAME: Dorothy Devine MR#: 55770

ATTENDING PHYSICIAN: L. Dacota, M.D. ADM: 5-5-XX

DISCH: 5-11-XX

HISTORY: The patient is a 53-year-old female with a long-standing history of diabetes and hypertension who was first seen by Dr. Dacota in October 1989, for severe hypertension and renal insufficiency and BUN of 32 and creatinine 2.1. The duration of diabetes was unclear to the patient. It was only known that the patient has had diabetes since 1987. The patient was seen approximately 1 week prior to admission for increasing dyspnea, PND, as well as cough, which was worse at night and productive at times as well. She has had some chilly sensations but denied any fevers. The patient was seen the day prior to admission by Dr. Schmidt and it was felt she was in mild congestive heart failure. Chest x-ray at that time also showed a right lower lobe infiltrate and the patient was started on erythromycin q. 6 hours and was continued on her diuretics as she was before. The patient was followed up the next day by Dr. Dacota. She complained of severe progressive dyspnea increasing PND over the previous week, fatigue, and weakness.

The patient stated that there was some mild improvement of her cough but the PND had not improved. It was felt that she should be admitted for further management.

At the previous visit to the clinic the patient was noncompliant with her follow-up. She has had progressive decline in her renal function and as of March 1992, her BUN was 85 and creatinine was 8.9. Because of this the patient was advised to consider dialytic treatment and this was stated to her 6 months prior to this time, but she postponed her decision and had felt that she did not want to go on hemodialysis. She was debating if peritoneal dialysis would be an alternative and was advised to see a surgeon for peritoneal dialysis catheter placement but failed to show up for any appointment. The patient is admitted now for therapy for her congestive heart failure and for Tenckhoff catheter placement.

PAST MEDICAL HISTORY: The patient has had two admissions for childbirth and had a D&C in 1975 and a knee operation in 1963.

MEDICATIONS: Her medications at the time of admission included Procardia XL 30 mg p.o. q. day, Catapres TTS patch 0.2 mg q. week, Capoten 50 mg p.o. b.i.d., Lasix 40 mg two tablets in the morning and one tablet in the afternoon, Zaroxolyn 2.5 mg p.o. b.i.d., and Micronase 2.5 mg p.o. three tablets in the morning before breakfast and two at dinner.

CASE 6

CASE SUMMARY (cont.)

SOCIAL HISTORY: The patient is a secretary in a dental office. She does not smoke or drink. She denies IV drug usage.

FAMILY HISTORY: Remarkable for diabetes in her father and grandmother and history of hypertension.

REVIEW OF SYSTEMS: Weakness, fatigue and dyspnea, leg edema, nausea and heartburn. The patient denies weight loss.

PHYSICAL EXAMINATION: She was a well-developed obese female with mild respiratory distress. Blood pressure 200/90 lying down without orthostatic changes. Heart rate 104. Respiratory rate 22. She was afebrile. HEENT exam revealed marked pallor with mild periorbital edema. There was no icterus. Her mucous membranes were moist. The fundi revealed diabetic retinopathy with hard exudates as well as proliferative retinopathy. The neck was remarkable for jugular venous distention at 30°. There were no carotid bruits or adenopathy. There was no thyromegaly. The lungs revealed bibasilar rales, right greater than left. Cardiovascular: PMI was at the 6th intercostal space, slightly left of the midclavicular line. It was tachycardic with an S^3 and a soft systolic murmur over the valvular areas. There was no rub. Her abdomen was soft, obese, without hepatosplenomegaly. There was no fluid wave. Extremities were without edema. There were 2+ pedal pulses bilaterally. There was no cyanosis or clubbing. Neurologic exam was nonfocal.

LABORATORY: Calcium 8.1, ionized calcium 1.9, phosphorus 5.5, glucose 289, uric acid 8.2. BUN 70, creatinine 7. Total protein 6, albumin 3.3, globulin 2.7, total bilirubin 0.4, SGPT 11, alkaline phosphatase 69, LDH 229, SGOT 11. Sodium 135, potassium 4.8, chloride 98. CO_2 22, triglycerides 314, cholesterol 247. Hepatitis B surface antigen was negative. PT, PTT were in control. Hemoglobin was 6.4, hematocrit 20.5. Platelet count 400. Her last creatinine clearance done 1-7-92, creatinine 6, 10 ml creatinine cleared per minute and total protein 10.24.

The ECG showed sinus tachycardia with nonspecific ST-T wave changes.

HOSPITAL COURSE: The patient was admitted with advancing chronic renal failure to end-stage renal disease secondary to diabetic nephropathy with nephrotic syndrome. Congestive heart failure class II. Anemia secondary to renal failure. Hypertension. The patient was admitted, had IV Lasix to improve her congestive heart failure and she was seen by Dr. Kevin Lori for PD catheter placement. The patient diuresed well. Her initial weight at the time of admission was 181. Her discharge weight is 171. The patient's blood sugars fluctuated during the time of her admission and her Micronase was decreased to 1.25 mg p.o. q. day with blood sugars ranging

CASE 6

CASE SUMMARY (cont.)

anywhere from 60 to 125. The patient had a Tenckhoff catheter placed on 4-7-19XX. There were no complications during her surgery. After her surgery, the patient had good bowel movements determined by the symptoms of flatus.

At the time of discharge her weight is 171. Blood pressure 120/70, pulse 86, respiratory rate 22, temperature 98. The patient's exam reveals clear lungs bilaterally. Cardiovascular is regular rate and rhythm with a II/VI systolic murmur without rub or gallop. Her abdomen is soft with normal bowel sounds with mild tenderness along her Tenckhoff catheter incision. Her extremities are without edema.

DISCHARGE LABS: BUN 97, creatinine 9.9, potassium 5.1, sodium 136, chloride 96, CO_2 24, WBC 10.1, hemoglobin 8.4, hematocrit 24.6, platelets 475, calcium 8.0, phosphorus 6.5, albumin 3.0.

DISCHARGE MEDS: Her medicines at the time of discharge include Colace 100 mg p.o. b.i.d., Tylenol #3 one p.o. q. 4–6 hours p.r.n. pain, dispense 15, erythromycin 333 mg one p.o. t.i.d. to be taken 7 more days to complete a 10-day course, Os-Cal 500 one p.o. with meals, Benadryl 50 mg p.o. q. h.s., Erythropoietin 4,000 units sub-cut Monday, Wednesday, and Friday, Lasix 80 mg p.o. b.i.d., Zaroxolyn 2.5 mg to be given 30 minutes prior to Lasix twice a day, Capoten 50 mg p.o. b.i.d., Catapres TTS patch 0.2 mg to be applied one time per week, Quinamm 200 mg p.o. q. h.s., Procardia XL 30 mg p.o. q. day.

The patient will be followed up at the clinic at the time of discharge to have a Tenckhoff catheter flushed and is to be seen by Dr. Dacota next week.

Jeff Green, M.D.

JG/LM

Case 6 Study Questions

1. This patient has diabetes, which is an endocrine disorder. How is this affecting at least two other body systems?
2. This patient chose peritoneal dialysis instead of hemodialysis. Describe the difference between the two forms of dialysis.
3. This patient is said to be without hepatosplenomegaly. What does this mean?
4. What does the abbreviation BUN mean? What type of test provides this information?
5. The report states that "At the previous visit to the clinic the patient was noncompliant with the follow-up." What does noncompliant mean?

CASE 7

CONSULTATION REPORT

PATIENT NAME: Bruce Jaeger   DATE: 8-8-XX

REF. PHYSICIAN: G. Plymouth, M.D.

Thank you very much for referring Bruce Jaeger to me. As you know, he is a 24-year-old gentleman who complains of red, mucousy, crusty eyes of approximately 1 week's duration. He has a history of daily soft contact lens wear. Significant findings include a recent cold.

Examination revealed a visual acuity of 20/25-2 in the right eye and 20/25-3 in the left eye. His pupils were equal, round, and reactive to light without any Marcus Gunn reaction. The external examination revealed no palpable preauricular nodes. His extraocular movements were intact. A detailed slit-lamp examination of the anterior segment revealed +1 to +2 conjunctival injection. The corneas exhibited numerous subepithelial infiltrates, more so on the right than the left eye. In addition, overlying superficial punctate staining was present. His anterior chambers were deep and quiet and the irises round. Applanation intraocular pressures were deferred. A fundus examination was benign.

In conclusion, Bruce does indeed have conjunctivitis of both eyes, apparently of the adenovirus (EKC) variety. I advised him about contagiousness and asked him to use Bleph-10 four times a day in both eyes to prevent a secondary infection. In addition, I have asked him to return in 2 weeks for a follow-up visit and to refrain from contact lens wear in the meantime. He will return to your care as soon as possible.

Thank you for your referral.

William Murphy, M.D.

WM/LM

Case 7 Study Questions

1. This patient has conjunctivitis of both eyes. What does this mean?
2. The doctor performed a slit-lamp examination. Briefly describe this procedure.
3. Find the eponym "Marcus Gunn reaction" in your medical dictionary. What heading was it listed under? What does it mean? Did you find more than one meaning for it?
4. Where are the preauricular nodes located? What kind of nodes are these?
5. Applanation intraocular pressures are measured with an applanation tonometer. Look this up in your medical dictionary. What heading was it listed under? How was this test described?

CASE 8

CONSULTATION REPORT

PATIENT NAME: Darryl McFadden   DATE: 5-4-XX

REF. PHYSICIAN: Steve Glass, M.D.

Thank you for referring the patient to me. His history is such that he complains of nasal blockage, postnasal drip, and cough especially at night. His symptoms are perennial, but mainly from March through October. He says he has been getting allergy injections for the past 5 years, but is not doing well.

His history sheet reveals that he is exposed to a feather pillow and also to dust and other factors in his household, and that seems to make him worse. He has been on Seldane medication, the only treatment he has had other than his injections.

The physical examination revealed the lungs were clear. There were no rales. There were decreased breath sounds on expiration, a little rhonchi. There was some nasal congestion of the turbinates, which were pale and engorged. There were no obvious pus pockets. There was a premaxillary edema bilaterally, especially on the right. There were some allergic shiners evident. There was some mild postnasal drip and there was some mild cervical lymphadenopathy. There was some slight tenderness over the epigastrium but no evidence of any masses or liver or spleen enlargement.

The patient also said he has been tested before by Burk Laboratory in 1987, and then apparently by IMS on molds alone in September 1990, none of which were remarkable. Allergy testing was done using scratch and intradermal, copies of which will be sent to you. On scratch, the patient showed allergy to several foods, primarily walnuts, milk, and chocolate. There was a definite allergy to trees, grasses, weeds, ragweed, and mold and also to feathers, house dust, mite dust, dog, and cat.

The patient also had a pulmonary function, which was unremarkable. Sinus x-rays failed to show any sinus disease. Nevertheless, there is still engorgement on clinical examination.

The patient was given a sample of Beconase AQ and instructed to use two sprays every 12 hours each nostril and to get more of this medication from his physician. He is to continue the Seldane, the same dose you have prescribed, as needed, and he is to receive allergy injections.

We should start probably twice a week as long as he can tolerate this, namely his arms getting sore or developing any other clinical symptoms of congestion from the shots. If he cannot continue, we will have to drop him back to once a week, which should be given for a year and then tapered down slowly to reach once a month for 3 years, if possible.

CASE 8

CONSULTATION REPORT (cont.)

Thank you for referring this patient. Vaccines will be sent to your office as well as the copies of other records on this patient.

Jerry Perlmutter, M.D.

JP/LM

Case 8 Study Questions

1. The report noted there were no rales. What are rales?
2. Mild cervical lymphadenophy was noted. What area was examined to find this? Which body system does it involve?
3. There was also some slight tenderness over the epigastrium. Where is this located?
4. What are the patient's primary food allergies?
5. What ongoing treatment was recommended for this patient?

CASE 9

CONSULTATION REPORT

PATIENT NAME: John Thomas   DATE: 4-5-XX

DIAGNOSES:
1. Benign paroxysmal positional vertigo, probably secondary to airplane crash.
2. Possible right temporal bone fracture, longitudinal type (not demonstrated by CT scan of August 7, 1991).

HISTORY: This 45-year-old patient was involved in an airplane crash when two airplanes crashed on a runway in December 1989. He states that he was hit with debris on the right side of his head and sustained several lacerations on the right side of his head and ear. He had no bleeding from the ear canal and no facial weakness. There was some numbness of the right ear canal, which was present for one week and then improved. The patient noted immediate hearing loss in the right ear after the accident, which has continued until this time. The patient was never unconscious. In addition, the patient has noted momentary vertigo when looking down since the accident, with the vertigo having improved slightly. He has some pressure in the right ear, which has persisted since the accident. The patient has episodes of dizziness at least once a day.

Ears, nose and throat examination revealed normal eardrums, with a healed laceration of the right auricle involving the helix. The nasal septum was deviated slightly to the right with increased mucus. Throat examination was negative.

An audiogram was obtained on July 24, 1991, at the time of the patient's initial visit. This audiogram revealed an average 13-dB hearing loss through the speech frequencies in the right ear with an average loss of 7 dB loss in the left ear. Speech discrimination was normal in both ears. There was a high-frequency loss of 25 dB in the right ear at 8000 cycles with only a 5-dB loss in the left ear at 8000 cycles. It was our impression that the patient had a very mild hearing loss of the right ear with excellent discrimination. An ABR (auditory brainstem response) was recommended, and this was performed also on July 24, 1991. The ABR was normal.

An ENG (electronyastagmography) was obtained on August 23, 1991, because of a history of vertigo. This test suggested vestibular pathology with possible CNS disorder due to optokinetic results. The patient was unable to perform tasks to the left and the optokinetic responses were unequal. A repeat audiogram on October 11, 1991, revealed average hearing loss of 23 dB in the right ear. A CT scan of the temporal bones was obtained on August 2, 1991, and was normal, except for some mucosal thickening of the sphenoid sinus.

The patient was treated initially with Nasalcrom nose spray for mild allergies and Antivert 12.5 mg three times a day for dizziness. At a follow-up visit on August 21, the patient stated that the light-headedness and dizziness persisted with no change in condition. He continued to have positional dizziness and mild hearing loss. At that time, the patient was given prescriptions for Seldane 60 mg b.i.d. and a displacement sinus procedure was performed in the office because of the mild sphenoid sinusitis.

IMPRESSION: The patient did have benign paroxysmal positional vertigo relating to the airplane accident. He also has a possible right temporal bone fracture, although this has not been demonstrated by the CT scan. In many cases temporal bone fractures are very small and of the longitudinal type and may not be apparent on CT scans.

Fortunately, the hearing loss is mild in the right ear and probably will not require a hearing aid. The prognosis for vertigo varies. The patient has a history of slightly elevated cholesterol, which may aggravate the dizziness somewhat. In addition, we ordered a 2-hour blood sugar with insulin levels to determine if other factors are contributing to his dizziness.

James Milligan, M.D.

JM/LM

Case 9 Study Questions

1. This patient is reported to be suffering from vertigo. What does this mean?
2. This is described as paroxysmal positional vertigo. What does paroxysmal mean? How does this relate to vertigo?
3. An electronyastagmography (ENG) was obtained. Which sense does an ENG test?
4. The optokinetic responses were unequal. What does optokinetic mean?
5. What is the prognosis for this patient with vertigo?

CASE 10

CONSULTATION REPORT

PATIENT NAME: Violet Hansen   MR#: 234889

ATTENDING PHYSICIAN: S. Manley, M.D.   ROOM#: 615

CONSULTING PHYSICIAN: David Wundermiser, M.D.

DATE OF CONSULTATION: 3-7-XX

REASON FOR CONSULTATION: Anemia and possible underlying autoimmune disease process.

HISTORY: This 56-year-old, delightful, black female, retired domestic worker since 1988, was seen and examined at the request of Dr. Manley for evaluation and treatment of anemia and possible underlying autoimmune disease.

IMPRESSIONS:

1. Normochromic, normocytic anemia (hemoglobin and hematocrit of 10.1/30.4 with MCV 91.2 as of 3-5-91), of chronic disease secondary to probable underlying rheumatoid arthritis. Rule out concomitant nutritional anemia secondary to malabsorption syndrome? Doubtful for hemolytic anemia but will rule it out.

2. Recurrent partial small bowel obstruction ever since cholecystectomy in January 1988, requiring surgical exploration in February 1988, with "hard fixed mesentery" grossly. Upper gastrointestinal dysmotility disorder, complicating bowel obstruction further. Rule out fibrosing peritonitis due to underlying collagen vascular disease?

3. "Arthritis" since August 1988, most likely rheumatoid arthritis as shown by bilateral symmetric ulnar deviation with PIP and MP joint involvement in both hands and early morning stiffness that loosens up toward the end of the day.

4. Health surveillance, status postcholecystectomy for symptomatic gallstones in January 1988, with "concrete-like bile" grossly. History of hypertension since 1969, but medications discontinued in 1988, due to side effects. Home TPN complicated by catheter sepsis and endocarditis in 1989 or 1990. Steady weight loss from her usual 150 to 160 pounds, prior to cholecystectomy which went down as low as 98 pounds, but now leveled off around 125 pounds. Rule out malabsorption syndrome. Nonsmoker, nondrinker, no known drug allergies. Nullipara with menarche at age 15 and menopause around age 32, on having D&C for irregular period. Retired, domestic worker until 1988.

CASE 10

CONSULTATION REPORT (cont.)

DISPOSITION AND RECOMMENDATIONS:

1. I took the liberty of ordering a lot of additional anemia and underlying collagen vascular work-ups. In addition to a CBC, sedimentation rate, rheumatoid factor, I added the G6PD, direct Coombs', SGPT, GGT, etc. PSH, serum ferritin, level will also be checked. For further evaluation of the collagen vascular disorder possibility, I ordered the entire RNP (ribonuclear protein), as well as anti-ENA (extractable nucleic acid) antibodies along with total complements and the hemolytic component will be checked.

2. I also took the liberty of ordering a serum protein electrophoresis with immuno-electrophoresis for B cells and the skin panel with intermediate PPD, Candida for T-cell immune function.

3. X-rays of both hands, wrists, and feet will be performed looking for clues for specific arthritis although rheumatoid arthritis is strongly suspected.

4. Will consider bone marrow aspiration and biopsy if current anemia continues to deteriorate and is unresponsive to hematinics which she has been on (Theragran N).

5. More diagnostic and therapeutic recommendations to follow after reviewing above initial data.

CLINICAL BACKGROUND: This is a fascinating, 56-year-old, black female, nulliparous, retired domestic worker since 1988, who was admitted on 3-4-91, with nausea, vomiting, and dehydration secondary to recurrent partial small-bowel obstruction. Her past medical history is significant for cholecystectomy for symptomatic gallstones in January 1988, by Dr. Agent. Within a month after surgery, the patient had to be re-explored in February 1988, mainly because of the bowel obstruction, although her postoperative course was complicated by "pneumonia."

Subsequent to this exploratory correction of the small-bowel obstruction, the patient had to be placed on home TPN through a central line; however, she developed catheter-associated sepsis, including endocarditis. Therefore, ultimately a central line had to be removed. She developed recurrent partial small bowel obstruction recently, requiring hospitalization here from 2-13-91 through 2-20-91. There appears to be a motility disorder of the GI tract, because the barium swallow has been persistently staying in the gastric region without moving further downward for long periods of time, according to the attending physician. She has been steadily losing weight from her usual 150 to 160 pounds prior to cholecystectomy, one time reaching to a low of 98 pounds, but now having regained to about 125 pounds.

Other pertinent past medical history is that of a severe "arthritis", which involved the right hip to the point that she was not able to walk around August 1988, and now is taking Naprosyn which has helped. She has been stiff in her fingers mostly on waking

CASE 10

CONSULTATION REPORT (cont.)

up in the morning, but generally stiffness and pain gradually subside as the day goes by. Like-wise, bilateral feet and toes are stiff and hurting also. Other pertinent medical history includes a history of hypertension diagnosed around 1969, requiring medication; however, in 1988, antihypertensive medication had to be stopped because of side effects.

Pertinent physical examination at this time shows a thin, emaciated black female but a delightful lady with full smiles on her face. She is fully alert and oriented. No scleral icterus but moderate conjunctival pallor. No significant lymphadenopathy around the neck, axilla, or groin, except for about 1 cm easily moveable, nontender, lymphadenopathy in the left axillary area. Chest clear. Heart normal sinus rhythm. No hepatosplenomegaly or any abdominal mass. No bound tenderness over the spine. No pitting edema or ecchymosis but most impressive is the bilateral symmetric ulnar deviation with lateral muscle wasting in the small fingers and palm, plus involvement of the PIP and MP joints, seen in both hands and wrists.

Pertinent laboratory data at this time show hemoglobin, hematocrit 10.1/30.4 with MCV 91.2, associated with a normal WBC count 5.1 (32% lymphs, 3% mono, and 65% granulocytes) and likewise normal platelet count of 208,000 on 3-5-91. Urinalysis was unremarkable except for 3-5 WBC/hpf and the SMA-7 so far shows no abnormality. Admission chest PA and lateral showed no active pulmonary disease but arteriosclerosis and admission flat plate of the abdomen showed changes consistent with a partial and presumably recurrent high small bowel obstruction probably at the level of the ligament of Treitz.

Thank you very much for this interesting and challenging consult opportunity. I will follow closely with you.

David Wundermiser, M.D.

Case 10 Study Questions

1. Dr. Manley wants to rule out malabsorption syndrome. What is malabsorption syndrome? Where did you find this information in your medical dictionary?
2. The reason for consultation includes possible underlying autoimmune disease process. What autoimmune disease is identified in the report?
3. There is mention of complications of home TPN. What does the abbreviation TPN mean?
4. The doctor ordered a Coombs' test. Look this test up in your medical dictionary? What heading was it listed under? What kind of specimen (blood, tissue, or urine) is required for this test?
5. Why was this patient admitted to the hospital this time?

CASE 11

CONSULTATION REPORT

PATIENT NAME: Mark Marvel   DATE: 4-4-XX

REF. PHYS.: Denise Dimpler, D.O.

This is a follow-up to our telephone discussion. The problems identified following the patient's diagnosis of AIDS include: (1) weight loss, (2) diarrhea, which he said is getting better, (3) elevated liver function tests. It is noted that he is a hepatitis B carrier, (4) productive cough, the etiology of which is not clear. Clinically, he seems to have a bronchitis and is coughing up what looks like mucous plugs. He does not have a fever. Other possibilities include PCP versus even tuberculosis. (5) He has a bad tooth, the last molar on the upper right, which appears to be carious, although not grossly infected at this time, in terms of abscess. (6) He has numbness of his feet.

On physical examination, generally, he appears in no apparent distress. He does have a persistent cough, productive of saliva mixed with thick gray-yellow mucous plugs. HEENT reveals what looks like dry skin involving his beard and nasolabial folds. The oral cavity is unremarkable except for the tooth. He does not have thrush at this time. I understand he is taking Diflucan. His neck is supple. No lymph nodes were palpated. The chest reveals diffuse scattered coarse rhonchi which changes with his cough. He has good air flow throughout. Cardiovascular reveals regular rate and rhythm. There is a very soft systolic murmur, Grade I-II/VI at the left sternal border. The abdomen is benign. The extremities are remarkable for one to two lymph nodes in both axilla which were about 0.5 cm in size, well circumscribed and nontender.

I received the labs that you sent with the patient and reviewed them. From 7-18-92, his CBC appears reasonable for him with a WBC of 3.1. Hemoglobin 12.6. Platelets 126,000. He tells me his AZT has been increased to five times a day, but it is not clear to me when that was done in relationship to these labs. His CMV titer has been consistently elevated on 7-18-92, 5-22-92, and 4-11-92. Hepatitis B surface antigen and hepatitis Be antigen have been positive with a negative hepatitis B surface antibody on 4-11-92, and 2-28-91, which suggests a carrier status. The stool studies, including culture, *Clostridium difficile* and ova and parasites are all negative from 6-9-92.

IMPRESSIONS:

1. Overall, he is apparently not doing as well as he has in the past. He has lost some weight and he has persistent cough, although he does not have frank shortness of breath or night sweats or persistent fever. He may improve in the general condition simply by elevating the dose of AZT.

CASE 11

CONSULTATION REPORT (cont.)

2. The cough should be worked up for PCP versus tuberculosis. I note that the routine sputum Gram stain and culture are still pending. The mucous plugs may suggest that he has an element of asthma and he may benefit from bronchodilators.

3. Peripheral neuropathy is most likely related to the HIV itself; because he has been on a low dose of AZT 300 mg a day, it is unlikely to be the cause of his problem specifically.

4. Hepatitis B carrier state. I discussed this with Mr. Vincent. He informs me that he has been celibate since his diagnosis of HIV.

5. With regard to his tooth, I suggest that he see a dentist. There are a number of dentists who will see HIV positive patients. I will refer you to the AIDS Consortium for a list of those.

PLAN:

1. Increase the AZT to five times a day. Monitor the CBC closely, and if necessary, the white count and his hemoglobin can be supported with Neupogen or Epogen, respectively. If you wish, we can make arrangements to instruct the patient in our day hospital to give these medications to himself. They are subcutaneous injections in the event they should be needed.

2. Work-up of his cough. Suggest sputum for AFB q. a.m. times 3. Sputum for silver stain to evaluate for PCP, as I discussed with you. Await Gram stain and culture of the sputum already sent and treat him with antibiotics according to the culture and sensitivity results. Suggest a follow-up chest x-ray.

3. The peripheral neuropathy may present a problem in terms of alternative therapy, i.e., DDI or DD, but that remains to be seen.

4. With regard to his elevated liver function test, it is difficult to say what the etiology may be. Of course, the hepatitis B may be playing a role. Alternatively, CMV may be part of the picture. If the liver function tests remain elevated or increase, suggest GI evaluation. He may need a liver biopsy to ultimately determine the etiology.

5. The diarrhea could have a number of causes as well. If it recurs, suggest stool for Cryptostoridium stain and if it persists, then the patient may need a colonoscopy to evaluate for other causes such as CMV.

CASE 11

CONSULTATION REPORT (cont.)

I left instructions with the patient to contact your office for the above work-up. If you have any questions, or if I can be of any further assistance, please do not hesitate to call me.

Sincerely,

Lois Lambert, D.O.

LL/LM

Case 11 Study Questions

1. Ronchi were mention in the chest examination. What does this mean? What kind of examination would reveal ronchi?
2. The report states, "He does not have thrush at this time." What is thrush? Why would it be expected that this patient might have it?
3. Impressions include "hepatitis B carrier state." What does this mean?
4. The report states, "CMV titer has been consistently elevated." What does the abbreviation CMV mean? What kind of specimen (blood, tissue, or urine) is required for this test?
5. Sputum tests are recommended. What is sputum?

CASE 12

CONSULTATION REPORT

January 16, 19XX

K. McAulay, M.D.
9925 San Roma Road
Masonville, FL 35525

RE: Leonard Mucini

Dear Dr. McAulay:

I first saw Mr. Leonard Mucini in my office on December 1, 1994. At that time he complained of decreased vision.

His best corrected visual acuity was 20/50-3 in the right eye and 20/40-3 in the left eye. He had a large myopic shift to his refraction. Biomicroscopic examination revealed bilateral nuclear sclerotic cataracts, the right being greater than the left. There were bilateral 360° synechiae with scattered KP. The fundus was difficult to observe because of dilation only to 3 mm. Intraocular pressures were found to be 22 mm Hg in each eye.

The patient was subsequently followed and when he returned on June 29, 1995, he complained of decreased vision. His visual acuity had decreased to 20/80 in the right eye. The remainder of the exam was the same.

Cataract surgery with intraocular lens implantation was fully discussed with Mr. Mucini. On July 16, an uneventful phacoemulsification of the right cataract with intraocular lens implantation was performed. The patient also had a radial iridotomy with 10-0 prolene repair and lysis of the synechia.

The patient did well postoperatively; however, when seen again on January 8, 1996, he had developed a clouded posterior capsule with precipitates on the anterior intraocular lens surface. A YAG posterior capsulotomy was performed and the anterior precipitates were also cleared at that time. The patient's vision cleared to 20/40; however, he subsequently developed more lens precipitates and required additional YAG laser treatments to remove the precipitates. Steroid drops were used to try and combat a recurrence of the lens precipitates.

The patient returned to see me on August 9. At that time he noted decreased vision in the left eye and desired cataract surgery with lens implantation. A similar surgical procedure was performed on the left eye on August 22. Again, the patient did well postoperatively.

CASE 12

CONSULTATION REPORT (cont.)

When last seen in the office on October 1, 19XX, the patient had a best corrected visual acuity of 20/30 in the right eye and 20/60 in the left eye. There was a mild posterior capsular haze, which was probably restricting his visual improvement in the left eye. A new glasses prescription was given to the patient and he was told to followup with an ophthalmologist when he moved to Florida.

If I can be of any further help, please feel free to contact me.

Sincerely yours,

Marvin Mitchell, M.D.

MM/LM

Case 12 Study Questions

1. The report describes "a large myopic shift." What does myopic mean?
2. Bilateral synechiae were found. What are synechiae?
3. Phacoemulsification was performed. What does this mean?
4. A YAG posterior capulotomy was performed? What major piece of equipment was used and how might a lay person describe this procedure.
5. The report notes the patient's corrected visual acuity. What does corrected visual acuity mean?

CASE 13

OPERATIVE REPORT

PATIENT NAME: Park, Dennis   MR#: 84321

SURGEON: P. Moylan, M.D.   ROOM#: 423A

PREOPERATIVE DIAGNOSIS: Recurrent lower GI bleeding

POSTOPERATIVE DIAGNOSIS: Sigmoid diverticulosis most likely the source of his lower GI bleeding, no evidence of malignancy or evidence of space-occupying lesion in the entire colon. No evidence of dysplasia.

PROCEDURES PERFORMED: Total colonoscopy

ANESTHESIA: IV Sedation

DESCRIPTION OF PROCEDURE: The patient was prepared for 2 days with clear liquids on an outpatient basis prior to his procedure early this morning. In the left lateral decubitus position, the patient was given intravenous glucagon through the IV tubing, followed by Valium 10 mg and Demerol 50 mg successively. The patient went into light sleep. The perianal and anal inspection with my forefinger did not reveal any significant findings. The fiberoptic colonoscope was inserted without any difficulty and by manipulating the tip of the scope, it was able to pass from the rectum to the rectosigmoid and to the sigmoid colon. There are multiple areas of diverticula in the rectosigmoid and sigmoid colon, and in the proximal part of the ascending colon. No evidence of a space-occupying lesion or malignancy in this area. There is some bleeding, but minimal in amount and not very active in the sigmoid colon. The scope was passed through the ascending colon up to the splenic flexure, transverse colon, hepatic flexure, and ascending colon to the cecum area. No evidence of abnormalities noted, except for few and occasional scattered diverticula in the colon, but predominantly in the sigmoid and rectosigmoid areas. The scope was gradually withdrawn and investigation from the cecal area down to the ascending, transverse, splenic and ascending colon, sigmoid and rectosigmoid and rectum, and no other abnormalities were noted except for the above description.

The patient tolerated the procedure well and since he developed mild hypertension, and local reaction from his intravenous medication, he was given Adrenalin 1:1,000 0.2 ml intravenously. He will be observed at the In and Out Recovery Room and will be discharged as soon as he is stabilized.

Peter Moylan, M.D.

PM/LM

Case 13 Study Questions

1. What procedure(s) were performed as described in this report.
2. What was the purpose of administering Valium and Demerol preoperatively.
3. What major piece of equipment was used for this examination?
4. The postoperative diagnosis was diverticulosis. What is diverticulosis?
5. The postoperative diagnosis indicated no evidence of dysplasia. What is dysplasia?

CASE 14

OPERATIVE REPORT

PATIENT NAME: Virginia Sloan   MR#: 45879

ATTENDING PHYSICIAN: Marjorie Wright, M.D.   ROOM#: 457

SURGEON: Penny Render, M.D.
ASSISTANT:

PREOPERATIVE DIAGNOSIS: Carcinoma of the urinary bladder secondary to CA of the colon. Anemia and hypokalemia.

POSTOPERATIVE DIAGNOSIS: Same.

PROCEDURES PERFORMED: Cystoscopy under local anesthesia.

ANESTHESIA: Local.

COMMENT: This 70-year-old woman has previously had a colon resection and partial cystectomy for primary carcinoma of the sigmoid colon that had perforated the bladder causing a fistula. At the present time, she is known to have a recurrence of an adenocarcinoma in the upper portion of the bladder. She has been hospitalized for dehydration and anemia and the opportunity is now taken to check the bladder even though a TUR of the bladder tumor cannot be performed as the serum potassium is only 3.2, making general anesthesia dangerous.

DESCRIPTION OF PROCEDURE: The patient was brought to the Cystoscopy Room. The external genitalia prepared with Septisol, sterile water and sterile drape. Then 2% Xylocaine jelly was instilled in the urethra for topical anesthesia. A cystoscopy was performed using a 17 French cystoscope, using a 30° lens. The urine was cloudy, and malodorous and a urine culture was taken. Inspection of the bladder revealed a necrotic tumor on the upper left posterior bladder wall. There were no bleeding areas noted so no fulgurations were necessary. The tumor was quite large, but did not involve the lower half of the bladder and the lower ureters are not involved. It is quite likely this patient has pulmonary metastases, as she previously has had a pleural effusion and is undergoing chemotherapy. No Mitomycin C was instilled in the bladder today at the patient's request, as she thinks this irritates the bladder, although it was previously instilled when the patient had a TUR of the bladder, which was the cause of her symptoms.

Penny Render, M.D.

Case 14 Study Questions

1. Why was this patient hospitalized?
2. According to this report, what procedures were performed?
3. The preoperative diagnosis included hypokalemia. What is hypokalemia?
4. A TUR of the bladder tumor could not be performed. What does this abbreviation mean?
5. The report notes that the patient probably has pulmonary metastases? What does this mean?

CASE 15

OPERATIVE REPORT

PATIENT NAME: Louise Mendiere   MR#: 887-98-62

ATTENDING PHYSICIAN: Alan Mason, M.D.   ROOM#: 525

SURGEON: Ellen Kay, M.D.
RESIDENT SURGEON: Dr. Green
ASSISTANT:

PREOPERATIVE DIAGNOSIS: Fracture, left proximal ulna with posterior radial head dislocation.

POSTOPERATIVE DIAGNOSIS: Fracture, left proximal ulna with posterior radial head dislocation.

PROCEDURES PERFORMED: Open reduction, internal fixation of the left ulna with tension band wiring with closed reduction of the left radius.

ANESTHESIA: General.

COMPLICATIONS: None.

ESTIMATED BLOOD LOSS: Minimal.

OPERATIVE MATERIAL: 18-Gauge K-wire, two 0.062-inch K-wires.

DESCRIPTION OF PROCEDURE: The patient was prepped and draped in sterile fashion. The tourniquet was inflated to 250 mm Hg and a posterior approach to the elbow was made via a straight longitudinal incision. This was taken down to the posterior ulna and olecranon. The fracture site was visualized. After elevating the periosteum with the periosteal elevator, the fracture site was noted to be in the proximal metadiaphysis of the ulna. The fracture hematoma was removed from the fracture site with a combination of irrigation and a small curet. The fracture was then reduced by longitudinal traction and pronation of the extremity. Reduction was held with point of reduction clamps. After reduction, the reduction was stabilized by inserting two 0.062 inch K-wires from the posterior olecranon into the medullary canal of the ulna across the fracture site.

After stabilization in this fashion, the point of reduction clamps were removed to assess stability. The fracture was noted to be reduced and there was some motion at the fracture site with flexion/extension and pronation supination. This motion was minimal; however, further stabilization was added by tension band wiring and using a

CASE 15

OPERATIVE REPORT (cont.)

2-mm drill bit, approximately 1.5 cm distal to the fracture site and a drill hole was made transversely through the ulna. An 18-gauge K-wire was passed through this drill hole with a figure-of-eight made posteriorly just proximal to the fracture site and the wire looped superior to the two protruding K-wires at the site of the olecranon. The wire was then twisted and tied down laterally. Radiographs taken at this time revealed anatomic reduction of the fracture as well as relocation of the radial head. The wires were further tightened and the 0.062 inch K-wires were bent and cut as were the 18-gauge wires. The K-wires were tapped into the posterior olecranon.

The wound was then irrigated. The fracture was closed with 0 Vicryl suture in a figure-of-eight stitch. The subcutaneous tissue was reapproximated using 2-0 Vicryl sutures in a simple stitch as well as 3-0 Vicryl sutures in a simple interrupted buried stitch. The skin was reapproximated using staples. The extremity was then cleaned and dressed and immobilized in a posterior long-arm splint, thus concluding the operative procedure.

Alan Mason, M.D.

Case 15 Study Questions

1. In lay terms, what bone was fractured and where on the bone did the fracture occur?
2. The periosteum was elevated. What is the periosteum?
3. A fracture hematoma was removed. What is a hematoma?
4. What diagnostic method was used to reveal the anatomic reduction of the fracture?
5. What external means was used to immobilize the fracture?

CASE 16

OPERATIVE REPORT

PATIENT NAME: Sally Kellman   MR#: 44598

ATTENDING PHYSICIAN: Robert Smith, M.D.   ROOM#: 327

PREOPERATIVE DIAGNOSIS: (1) Pregnancy, uterine, nondelivered at 40+3 weeks estimated gestational age, (2) arrest of dilation.

SURGEON: Randy Chornack, M.D.
ANESTHETIST: Dr. Androsini
ANESTHESIA: Continuous lumbar epidural

MATERIAL FORWARDED TO THE LABORATORY FOR EXAMINATION: Umbilical cord blood gases

OPERATION PERFORMED: Lower primary cesarean section with Pfannenstiel skin incision and low transverse cervical uterine incision

INDICATIONS FOR SURGERY: The patient is a 17-year-old white female, G1 P0, last menstrual period May 24, who presented at 40+3 weeks estimated gestational age in early active labor. The patient had progressed through the transition phase at which time an intrauterine pressure catheter was placed due to difficulty assessing contractions on the external monitor. She progressed to 6 cm with fetal vertex at 0 station and in the occiput anterior position. She was contracting every 2 to 3 minutes with contractions that were 64, representative of adequate labor. She had an episode of bradycardia to the 80s lasting approximately 10 to 12 minutes, which responded to resuscitative measures including positioning and application of oxygen with a return to a baseline of 160s with some hypervariability; however, no further decels. In the face of adequate spontaneous labor and failure to progress beyond 6 cm for a period of 2 and 1/2 hours, decision was made to proceed to primary cesarean delivery.

FINDINGS: The patient was delivered of a liveborn female infant with Apgars of 9 and 9 and weight of 3422 g. Cord blood gases revealed an arterial pH of 7.27 and venous pH of 7.29.

DESCRIPTION OF OPERATION: In the OR under continuous lumbar epidural, the patient was prepped and draped in the usual fashion for cesarean delivery including sterile insertion of Foley catheter. She was placed in the supine position with a right hip role. A Pfannenstiel skin incision was made and carried down to the level of the rectus fascia, which was incised sharply and extended laterally. The rectus fascia was dissected off the underlying muscles, which were then separated in the midline and the peritoneal cavity was entered. The visceroperitoneum overlying the lower uterine segment

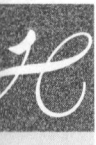

CASE 16

OPERATIVE REPORT (cont.)

was elevated and incised, and the bladder was dissected away from the lower uterine segment. A low transverse cervical incision was made and was extended with the bandage scissors. The amniotic cavity was entered, revealing moderate meconium. The fetal vertex was palpated, elevated and delivered. The baby was suctioned on the maternal abdomen. The remainder of the infant was delivered. The cord was doubly clamped and cut. The infant was passed up to the pediatricians in attendance. The placenta was manually extracted intact. It was a three-vessel cord. Pitocin and 2 g Ancef were added to the IV fluid after delivery of the placenta. The uterus was exteriorized and the uterine incision was examined. There was found to be a right inferolateral extension. There was also noted to be dissection in the myometrial layers of the lower uterine segment where a venous sinus had been entered with copious bleeding. This was controlled with interrupted figure-of-eight sutures and reapproximation of the myometrial layers. Closure of the right inferolateral extension incorporated the right uterine artery in the repair. This was closed in a running locking fashion with #1 chromic suture. The remainder of the uterine incision was likewise closed in a running locking fashion with #1 chromic suture. Good hemostasis was obtained. The bladder flap was then approximated using a running stitch of 2-0 chromic suture. The abdominal cavity was thoroughly irrigated and suctioned free of clots. The uterus was returned to the abdominal cavity and the pericolic gutters were then thoroughly irrigated. The parietal peritoneum was closed with 2-0 chromic in a running fashion. The fascia was then approximated using 0 Vicryl in a running fashion. The subcutaneous tissues were thoroughly irrigated and found to be hemostatic. The skin was closed with staples and sterile dressing was applied. The patient left for the recovery room in stable condition. She received 2400 ml of lactated Ringer's interoperatively and had 125 ml of urine output. Estimated blood loss was 1000 ml.

The patient tolerated the procedure well. There were no complications except the above-noted incisional extensions.

ADDENDUM: The pediatricians suctioned the infant postpartum, revealing no meconium below the cord.

Randy Chornack, M.D.

Case 16 Study Questions

1. Note the number of weeks of gestational age. Is this baby premature?
2. The patient experienced an episode of bradycardia. What is bradycardia and how long did this episode last?
3. The amniotic cavity contained meconium. What is meconium?
4. What methods were used to close the parietal peritoneum and the skin?
5. The baby's Apgars were 9 and 9. What are Apgars and what are the highest scores the baby could have received?

CASE 17

OPERATIVE REPORT

PATIENT NAME: Jack Jones   **MR#:** 33333   **DATE:** 4-7-XX

ATTENDING PHYSICIAN: M. Snyder, M.D.   **ROOM #:** 417B

PREOPERATIVE DIAGNOSIS: Left lower extremity femoral artery occlusion

SURGEON: Dr. Mills

FIRST ASSISTANT: Dr. Borland
SECOND ASSISTANT:

ANESTHETIST: Dr. Pes

ANESTHESIA:

TIME BEGAN: **TIME ENDED:**

CIRCULATING NURSE(S):

SCRUB NURSE(S):
TIME OPERATION BEGAN: **TIME OPERATION ENDED:**

OPERATIVE DIAGNOSIS: Same as above

DRAINS: 16 French Fley to the urinary bladder
SPONGE COUNT: Verified

OPERATION PERFORMED: Left femoral artery bypass

INDICATIONS FOR SURGERY: The patient is a 62-year-old male with progressive claudication, who on arteriogram, had an isolated obstruction of his left femoral artery at the common femoral region with good collateral blood flow. He had a past medical history of fem-pop disease with two femoral-popliteal bypasses. On his arteriogram, the femoral-popliteal bypass was also occluded; however, he had developed collateral flow with good reconstitution of the above-knee popliteal artery. His profunda femoral artery was very large secondary to collateral blood supply.

DESCRIPTION OF OPERATION: The patient was taken to the OR where, after adequate general anesthesia was rapidly obtained, he was prepped and draped in the usual manner. An incision was created in the left groin which extended on to the abdominal cavity and then curved laterally. This incision went distally down to approximately the proximal third of his thigh. The proximal portion of the wound was identified first and a retroperitoneal approach was used to gain access and control of his common femoral artery. The inguinal ligament had to be divided to facilitate this dissection. The ureter was identified easily and the common femoral artery was identified at a point proximal to the obstructed area. A good pulse was felt in this artery and it was encircled with two vascular loops for control.

CASE 17

OPERATIVE REPORT (cont.)

Attention was then directed toward the distal portion where the profunda femoral artery was identified deep in its muscular cavity and this was carefully dissected free of the vein and encircled with vascular loops as well. Having fully identified these two arterial segments, and having allowed for a graft between them, the patient was given 5000 units of heparin IV bolus by the anesthesiologist. Once this had been in and circulating for a couple of minutes, the umbilical tapes at the proximal portion were left untied; however, the distal segment was occluded. An arteriotomy was created with an 11 blade knife and extended with Potts scissors. The distal portion of the previously cut 6-mm vascular Dacron graft was then sutured in place using 6-0 Prolene. This was done in a running manner from the site of the graft around the heel and the toe back to the other side of the graft. The sutures were then left open and black-bleeding was confirmed. This was then tied. The graft itself was then flushed with heparinized saline solution, placed through the previously made tunnel in the region of the inguinal canal and the proximal portion was aligned carefully with the common femoral artery. At this point, an end of graft to side of common femoral artery anastomosis was undertaken after an arteriotomy was created with the 11 blade again. This was undertaken with 6-0 Prolene once again and sutured in a running manner. At the completion of the case, the patient had good pulsatile flow throughout the graft and had a distal pulse in his lower extremity where before he had not had one.

The wounds were very carefully examined for hemostasis and then closed in three layers with absorbable suture material. The patient had received preoperative antibiotics. The skin was closed with stainless steel staples. The patient was returned to the recovery room in stable condition.

Steven Mills, M.D.

SM/LM

Case 17 Study Questions

1. The patient suffered from progressive claudication. What is claudication?
2. What diagnostic study was mentioned as an indication for surgery?
3. Is this the first time the patient has had this type of surgery? If not, how many pervious surgeries are mentioned in his past medical history.
4. Heparin was administered during the surgery. Was this administered to prevent bleeding?
5. This was described as a heparin bolus and was administered by the anesthesiologist. Was this intravenous or gas administration? Was it administered slowly or all at once?

CASE 18

OPERATIVE REPORT

PATIENT NAME: Roberta Smiley   **MR#:** 35958

ATTENDING PHYSICIAN: M. Tillman, D.O.   **ROOM#:** 417

SURGEON: S. Wellman, D.O.

PREOPERATIVE DIAGNOSIS: Wilms' tumor of the left kidney.

OPERATIVE DIAGNOSIS: Wilms' tumor left kidney.

OPERATION PERFORMED: (1) Left nephrectomy, (2) left lymphadenectomy, (3) right external jugular dual lument broviac catheter, (4) inversion appendectomy.

INDICATIONS FOR SURGERY: The patient is a 2-year-old white female with an incidentally identified abdominal mass. Preoperative evaluation was consistent with a Wilms' tumor.

DESCRIPTION OF OPERATION: The patient was brought to the OR, where, after adequate general anesthesia was readily obtained, the region of her right neck was prepped and draped in the usual manner. An incision was created over the external jugular vein and extended down to the subcutaneous tissue with a knife. Via blunt and sharp dissection, the external jugular vein was identified and encircled with two silk ties. A venotomy was created and a Broviac catheter that had been previously tunneled through the skin, was placed through the vein and then under fluoroscopic guidance, was directed toward the superior vena cava. Positions having been confirmed with fluoroscopy, the catheter was sutured in place at the skin exit site and the skin was then closed with interrupted Vicryl sutures. These were subcuticular sutures. A sterile drape was then placed over the catheter itself. At this point, the abdomen was prepped and draped in the usual manner and all surgeons and equipment were changed in the way of gowns and gloves.

A transverse abdominal incision was created and carried down through the skin and subcutaneous tissues with cautery. The underlying muscle and fascia were divided with cautery as well. On entering the abdomen, appropriate retractors were placed, particularly a Richardson retractor in the left upper quadrant. The transverse colon and mesocolon were draped over the patient tumor mass, as was the sigmoid colon. After sharp dissection was undertaken, the sigmoid colon was reflected from left to right and very carefully dissected off of the superior aspect of the tumor. Via very careful blunt and sharp dissection, the left kidney was identified throughout its extent. The right kidney was also identified and very carefully explored before the left kidney was explored. There was no gross evidence of any injury or any tumor burden in the right kidney, i.e., the right kidney was normal. The left kidney was then mobilized as previously discussed, and via blunt

CASE 18

OPERATIVE REPORT (cont.)

dissection was developed up to its vascular pedicle. The renal artery and vein were individually ligated and divided. Suture ligatures were placed in the vessels as well. The left kidney and tumor mass were resected en bloc and the left adrenal gland was left in place.

Attention was then directed toward the renal fossa and a left-sided lymphadenectomy was undertaken throughout this region with resection of all gross lymph nodes. Having completed this, a warm pack was placed in this region and the appendix itself was identified. The mesoappendix was divided and ligated and stripped from the appendix and the appendix itself was then inverted on itself, after purse-string sutures had been placed around the appendiceal base. A suture ligature of 0 chromic was then placed around the appendiceal stump and the appendix itself was inverted and sutured in place with the previously placed purse-string GI silk suture. The left upper quadrant was again examined for hemostasis, which was found to be intact. The abdominal muscles were then closed in three separate layers using running and interrupted Vicryl sutures. The linea alba was reapproximated with figure of eight 2-0 Dexon sutures.

The skin was closed with a combination of stainless steel staples and steristrips. The patient tolerated the procedure very well. Blood loss was approximately 40 ml and the patient was taken to the Intensive Care Unit in stable condition.

S. Wellman, D.O.

Case 18 Study Questions

1. Look Wilms' tumor up in your medical dictionary. What was it listed under? What kind of tumor is it?
2. A nephrectomy was performed. What is a nephrectomy?
3. A venotomy was performed. What is a venotomy?
4. What diagnostic method was used to determine that the Broviac catheter was in the proper position?
5. A left-sided lymphadenectomy was performed. Why do you think this procedure was necessary?

CASE 19

OPERATIVE REPORT

PATIENT NAME: Milly Wilm   **MR#:** 123579

ATTENDING PHYSICIAN: R. Smart, M.D.   **ROOM#:** 358

PREOPERATIVE DIAGNOSIS: Right breast carcinoma

POSTOPERATIVE DIAGNOSIS: Same

SURGEON: David Boyle, M.D.

ANESTHESIA: General endotracheal with Forane nitrous

DRAINS: Two Jackson Pratt 7 mm to right breast

MATERIAL FORWARDED TO THE LABORATORY FOR EXAMINATION: Apical lymph node and right breast and axillary contents

OPERATION PERFORMED: Right modified radical mastectomy

DESCRIPTION OF OPERATION: With the usual sterile prep and drape, incision was made in curvilinear fashion superior and inferior to the right nipple from the sternoclavicular junction and laterally and superiorly for approximately 6–8 cm lateral to the nipple. This included the previously superior medial biopsy site. The flaps were then developed using Bovie electrocautery, Metzenbaum scissors until the breast tissue was dissected down to the chest wall superiorly to the clavicular junction and medially to the sternum inferiorly to the sixth rib and laterally to the anterior border of the latissimus dorsi. After the complete borders of the breast were obtained, the fascia overlying the pectoralis major was then incised and reflected inferiorly. This was done in a step-wise fashion using Metzenbaum scissors until the axillary contents from the axillary vein down and inferiorly anterior to the anterior border of the latissimus dorsi and medially to the chest wall. The cords in this region were dissected free easily inferiorly and medially taking care not to disturb the thoracodorsal nerve or the long thoracic nerve of Bell. Due to the patient's paralyzed state, we were unable to actually confirm the muscular activity associated with testing both of these nerves. However, we felt that we were clear of that throughout the dissection. After the axillary dissection was completed inferiorly and medially, the axillary contents and the breast were removed using Bovie electrocautery and Metzenbaum scissors. Hemostasis was accomplished using Bovie electrocautery as well as 3-0 Vicryl ties. A single apical axillary lymph node was also removed and a medium-sized clip was placed at that location. At that point, the breast and the axillary contents were removed en bloc and removed from the field. At that point, approximately 500 ml warm sterile water was

CASE 19

OPERATIVE REPORT (cont.)

used to irrigate the wound x two. After adequate hemostasis was ensured, two 3-0 Vicryl sutures were placed on the lateral aspect of the wound bringing the flap to the superficial fascia overlying the serratus anterior.

After this closure, two drains were then placed inferiorly, one into the axillary wall and one near the skin flap on the anterior chest. Each was hooked up to suction for the remainder of the case. The subcutaneous tissue was then closed using approximately twelve 3-0 Vicryl subcutaneous fashion. This was followed by a running subcuticular 3-0 Vicryl to close the skin. A sterile dressing was then applied over the wound and drain dressings were applied over the two drains. At that point, nonpressurized adhesive tape was placed over the sterile dressing.

The patient tolerated the procedure without difficulty and was extubated in the OR. There were no postoperative complications. The patient was transferred to the gurney and taken to the Recovery Room in good condition.

David Boyle, M.D.

Case 19 Study Questions

1. What was the preoperative diagnosis?
2. What operation was performed?
3. What is hemostasis? How was it accomplished?
4. What two forms of instrumentation were used to actually remove the breast?
5. The terms superior, inferior, lateral and medial are used to describe the incision. What do these terms mean? Based on the information in the report describe approximately where the incision was made.

CASE 20

DISCHARGE SUMMARY

NAME OF PATIENT: Peterson, Ron   **MR#:** 44582

DATE OF ADMISSION: 2-26-91

DATE OF DISCHARGE: 3-5-91

ATTENDING PHYSICIAN: E. Margolis, M.D.

FINAL DIAGNOSIS: Status post-exploratory laparotomy with colostomy for colostomy closure.

OPERATIVE PROCEDURE: 2-27-91, Colostomy closure, incidental appendectomy and enterolysis.

HISTORY: This is a history of a 21-year-old male who was admitted electively for a colostomy closure. The patient had sustained a gunshot wound about a month prior, which caused multiple holes in the small bowel, transecting anteriorly the rectum and its entirety with some spillage and the bladder. The small bowel was repaired primarily with one area that required resection. The colon was resected, the distal end dropped and the proximal brought out through the colostomy and the bladder was repaired primarily. The patient is being admitted for reconstitution of the GI tract. The past history otherwise is insignificant.

HOSPITAL COURSE: The patient underwent a bowel prep the first day of hospitalization. He was taken to surgery the second day of hospitalization where the colostomy was closed. An incidental appendectomy was also performed at this time. The patient's course was untoward. He was started on a clear liquid diet, the second day after surgery and gradually moved up. He learned how to do his own wound care of the colostomy site and he improved to the point that at the time of discharge he was on a regular diet, no IVs and ambulatory for 24 hours.

The patient has had good GI function. He will be seen in my office in 1 week.

_____
E. Margolis, M.D.

Case 20 Study Questions

1. Why had a colostomy been performed on this patient?
2. One of the operative procedures was enterolysis. What is enterolysis?
3. An incidental appendectomy was also performed. What does "incidental appendectomy" mean?
4. Before discharge the patient had been ambulatory for 24 hours. What does this mean?
5. The term laparotomy is used in the final diagnosis. Look laparotomy up in your medical dictionary. Did you find more than one definition? Which one do you think correctly applies here?

CASE 21

DISCHARGE SUMMARY

PATIENT NAME: Anthony Blacksmith   MR#: 13579

ATTENDING PHYSICIAN: Heather Dixon, M.D

DATE OF ADMISSION: DATE OF DISCHARGE:

DISCHARGE DIAGNOSES:

1. Sigmoid diverticulitis.

HISTORY OF PRESENT ILLNESS: The patient is a 43-year-old white male with a 12-day history of painless diarrhea associated with intermittent fever, chills, and left lower quadrant pain. The pain was diffuse at first, but the patient has had no pain now for the past 7 days prior to admission. He has been tolerating a regular diet. He was seen with the above symptoms and orthostasis. The pulse went from 54 to 104 from supine to a standing position.

He was treated with hydration and stool cultures were checked in the Emergency Room here. He was seen in the Emergency Room again with a temperature of 99.8 and a white cell count of 27,000. Differential was 86 segs and 6 bands. The patient was sent home with a diagnosis of diarrhea. He returned to the Emergency Room on the day of admission without improvement. White cell count was 29.8 with 86 segs and 8 bands. He was referred to the Gastroenterology Service where a flexible sigmoidoscopy was done, which showed purulent discharge from a sigmoid diverticulum. At the time of admission, the patient denied nausea, vomiting, melena, bloody stools, colicky pain, any abdominal pain at this time. His only complaint on admission was the diarrhea, fever, and chills.

PAST MEDICAL HISTORY: Significant for an L-5–S-1 herniated nucleus pulposus.

PAST SURGICAL HISTORY: The patient had a right inguinal herniorrhaphy in 1987. The patient denies the use of alcohol or tobacco.

MEDICATIONS: The patient only takes Motrin p.r.n.

ALLERGIES: The patient has no known drug allergies.

REVIEW OF SYSTEMS: Noncontributory.

PHYSICAL EXAMINATION: Temperature on admission was 100.9. Pulse 68. Respirations 12. Blood pressure 138/82. HEENT exam: the pupils were regular, round, and reactive to light and accommodation. Extraocular motions were intact. The sclera were clear. The mouth was clear. The neck was supple without masses. The lungs were clear bilaterally. The heart was regular rate and rhythm without murmur. Normal S^1 and S^2, negative JVD. The abdomen was round, soft. Bowel sounds mild. Left lower quadrant pain. Tenderness to deep palpation. There were no masses or rebound. No tenderness on pelvic shake or Hill test. There is no Rovsig sign. Rectal

CASE 21

DISCHARGE SUMMARY (cont.)

exam was deferred because the patient has just been status post flexible sigmoidoscopy. Extremities without edema, cyanosis, or clubbing. Neurologic exam was nonfocal.

LABORATORY EXAM: The patient had a Chem-1 sodium 140, potassium 4.4, chloride 101, bicarb 22, BUN 12, glucose 82, creatinine 0.9. Chem-2 showed AST 41, ALT 28, alkaline phosphatase 85, total bilirubin 0.9, LDH 1133. Chem-3, total protein 6.7, albumin 2.9, calcium 8.6, phosphorus 3.8, uric acid 5.8. Amylase 38. White cell count 29.8, hemoglobin 13.1, hematocrit 38.1, platelets 442. Differential showed 8 bands, 86 granulocytes, 2 lymphocytes, 4 monocytes.

HOSPITAL COURSE: The patient was admitted to the General Surgery Service and was placed on triple antibiotics with ampicillin, gentamicin, and clindamycin for approximately 7 days. On hospital day number 3, the patient's fever defervesced and his bowel movements started to become normal. All stool cultures and stool for O&P were all negative. He continued to do well on triple antibiotics and on house day number 7, antibiotics were stopped and the patient was placed on oral antibiotics, with Bactrim and Flagyl. The patient remained afebrile and on hospital day number 9 he was discharged home.

DISPOSITION: The patient is discharged home in good condition.

DISCHARGE MEDICATIONS: Metamucil one tbsp in juice p.o. q. a.m.; Bactrim double strength, one p.o. b.i.d. for 10 days and Flagyl 500 mg p.o. t.i.d. for 10 days. The patient was also instructed to continue a diet high in fiber. He has no other dietary restrictions.

FOLLOW-UP: The patient will follow up with the General Surgery Clinic in approximately 10–14 days, or sooner if he has any recurrence of the diarrhea, fever, chills, or abdominal pain.

Heather Dixon, M.D.

Case 21 Study Questions

1. The discharge diagnosis is sigmoid diverticulitis. Describe diverticulitis and state where it occurred in this patient.
2. Past surgical history includes a herniorrhaphy. What is a herniorrhaphy?
3. During the patient's hospital course his fever defervesced. What does this mean?
4. In the history of the patient's present illness, the term orthostasis is used. Look orthostasis up in your medical dictionary. If you cannot find it, seek out closely related terms (such as orthostatic). Based on this definition, and the information in the history, what do you think orthostasis means?
5. All stool cultures were negative for O&P. What does the abbreviation O&P mean?

CASE 22

DISCHARGE SUMMARY

PATIENT NAME: Dorothy Ryder   **MR#:** 58-96-42

ATTENDING PHYSICIAN: Morris Early, M.D.

ADMISSION DATE: **DISCHARGE DATE:**

ADMISSION DIAGNOSIS:
1. Multiple compression fractures of T-12, L-1, L-2 and L-4.

DISCHARGE DIAGNOSIS: Same as above, nonacute fractures.

HISTORY OF PRESENT ILLNESS: This is a 60-year-old female with a long history of multiple fractures dating back to 1962. She has a history of significant osteoporosis, which was diagnosed in 1991. The patient also has a history of osteoarthritis and had a right total hip replacement in 1988. The patient was in her usual state of health until approximately 2 days prior to admission when she stepped down in her living room, one step, and developed some backache. This became progressively worse over the next 2 days to the point where she was having difficulty ambulating and she presented to the Emergency Room.

On evaluation in the Emergency Room, it was noted that she had compression fractures of T-12, L-1, L-2, L-3 and L-4. However, these could not be ruled out as new or old fractures due to lack of previous x-rays in this area. The patient was admitted for further evaluation.

PAST MEDICAL HISTORY: The patient is retired and lives in a self-care apartment in a retirement community in Pine Valley. She does not smoke and has no alcohol intake. She takes Macrodantin one p.o. q. h.s. and calcium one t.i.d. She has been on a regular diet. She has had osteoporosis and osteoarthritis. Also of note is that approximately 10 days prior to admission, the patient sustained a left distal radius fracture for which she was treated with a splint by a civilian orthopedist.

PHYSICAL EXAMINATION: This is a well developed, well nourished elderly white female in no acute distress. She had moderate discomfort on movement. Her HEENT exam was essentially normal. Her lungs were clear. Heart had a regular rate and rhythm. Abdomen was soft and nontender. Her rectal showed good tone. Her back showed moderate tenderness to palpation in the upper lumbar and lower thoracic area. Neurologically, she was completely normal with cranial nerves being intact. Motor was 5/5 in all extremities, except for the left extremity, which was not examined secondary to her being in a splint. She had deep tendon reflexes 2+ and equal. Her sensory exam was normal.

CASE 22

DISCHARGE SUMMARY (cont.)

HOSPITAL COURSE: The patient was admitted and on the day following admission, she had a bone scan which revealed moderate DJD of the T&L spine with no evidence of acute compression fractures. The patient was placed on bed rest and was started with physical therapy and ambulation with which she has steadily progressed with decreasing pain and tenderness. The patient is now ambulating with a walker with a platform for her cast. Two days after admission her splint was changed to a long arm cast. Postcasting films showed no change in fracture alignment. The films were read by the hand team, which compared with the casting treatment, despite some slight loss of radiostyloid height.

Social Services and Physical Therapy were consulted. She is ambulating well with her walker and it is felt she will do well staying with members of her family over the next 10-14 days, after which time she will be able to go back to living in her apartment.

The patient will follow up with the Orthopedic Clinic in 10-14 days. She will follow up with her private physician for a distal radius fracture on discharge.

DISCHARGE MEDICATIONS: Tylenol #3, one or two p.o. q 4-6 h. p.r.n.; Macrodantin 50 mg p.o. q. h.s. and she will continue with her calcium t.i.d.

Morris Early, M.D.

Case 22 Study Questions

1. What are compression fractures?
2. The bone scan revealed moderate DJD. What does this abbreviation mean?
3. What had happened to this patient 10 days before this hospital admission?
4. This patient has had a joint replacement. What joint was replaced and when?
5. What diagnosed disorder was the primary cause of these compression fractures?

CASE 23

DISCHARGE SUMMARY

PATIENT NAME: Martin LaBlanc MR#: 45789

ATTENDING PHYSICIAN: Robert Malagwa, M.D.

DATE OF ADMISSION: DATE OF DISCHARGE:

DISCHARGE DIAGNOSES:
1. Left lower lobe pneumonia, viral versus bacterial, resolving.
2. Status post right upper lobe lobectomy, March 1989.
3. History of tobacco abuse.
4. History of posttraumatic seizures.

HISTORY OF PRESENT ILLNESS: This is a 67-year-old white male with a 1-day history of fever, myalgia, and dry cough. He denied shaking, chills, sputum production, chest pain, hemoptysis. He also denied history of pulmonary embolism and denied increasing shortness of breath, headache, neck stiffness, or abdominal discomfort.

PAST MEDICAL HISTORY: Significant for prolonged hospitalization for bronchiolitis obliterans with necrotizing pneumonia requiring intubation and subsequent right upper lobe lobectomy. His course was complicated by bronchial pole fistula. The patient also has a history of posttraumatic seizure in 1965, and a history of tobacco abuse of approximately 100 pack-years.

MEDICATIONS: On admission, medications were prednisone 5 mg p.o. q. day, multivitamins one a day, calcium carbonate one twice a day, Actifed inhaler four puffs q. 4 hours, albuterol inhaler three puffs q. 4 hours.

PHYSICAL EXAMINATION: Revealed an alert male in no acute distress. Temperature was 97.5, pulse 86 and regular. Respirations 22. Blood pressure 146/76. Physical examination was significant for dry rales of the left base with dullness to percussion and increased tactile fremitus. There were distant breath sounds bilaterally without wheezes or rhonchi. Heart was regular without murmurs, rubs or gallops. Extremities revealed no clubbing, cyanosis or edema.

Admission laboratory studies were significant for a WBC of 22.1 with 71% segs, 6% bands, 14% lymphs, 5% monos. Arterial blood gases on room air showed pH 7.39, PO_2 60, PCO_2 30. Chest x-ray showed right basilar and apical scarring with chronic surgical changes and chronic volume loss on the right. There appeared to be a new left lower lobe density without evidence of frank consolidation.

HOSPITAL COURSE: The patient was admitted for treatment of a presumed left lower lobe pneumonia. During this admission, he at no time produced sputum. Blood

CASE 23

DISCHARGE SUMMARY (cont.)

cultures were drawn and have shown no growth. The patient received three days of treatment with cefuroxime 1.5 g IV q. 8 hours, after which time he was switched to Ceftin 250 mg p.o. b.i.d. The patient has remained afebrile throughout his hospital course and now feels back to his baseline at the time of discharge.

DISCHARGE MEDICATIONS: Prednisone 5 mg p.o. q. day x 7 days; calcium carbonate one p.o. b.i.d., multivitamin one p.o. q. day; Actifed inhaler four puffs q. 4 hours; Albuterol inhaler three puffs q. 4 hours, and Ceftin 250 mg b.i.d. x 6 days. This will complete 10 full days of antibiotics.

The patient will call the Pulmonary Clinic for routine follow-up. He will call me in the Internal Medicine Clinic in the interim if any problems develop.

Robert Malagwa, M.D.

Case 23 Study Questions

1. The patient complained of myalgia. What is myalgia?
2. The patient denied experiencing hemoptysis. What is hemoptysis?
3. The patient's medical history includes a right upper lobe lobectomy. What is a lobectomy?
4. As stated in the hospital course, why was this patient admitted to the hospital?
5. During his hospitalization the patient was treated with cefuroxime. How was this administered?

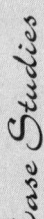

CASE 24

DISCHARGE SUMMARY

PATIENT: Martha Wembly   MR#: 445577

DATE OF ADMISSION: DATE OF DISCHARGE:

DISCHARGE DIAGNOSES:
1. Ventricular tachycardia.
2. Atherosclerotic heart disease.
3. Prolonged sinus pauses.
4. Diabetes mellitus.
5. Hypertension.
6. Hypothyroidism.
7. Hyperlipidemia.

HISTORY: This is a 71-year-old female who was brought into the hospital after ventricular tachycardia complicated a treadmill test in the office on the day of admission. There was also some minimal hypoglycemia with blood sugar near 50 and the symptoms transiently improving after some 50% dextrose was administered, but because the patient was still feeling slightly off she was admitted. The patient's history includes: high blood pressure, hypothyroidism, hypercholesterolemia, coronary artery disease status post microinfarction and recent PTCA.

Family history is significant for atrophic vaginitis. Mitral regurgitation. History of cataract extraction.

PHYSICAL EXAMINATION: Physical examination revealed a healthy appearing lady who appeared her stated age. Vital signs were normal with blood pressure 140/70. There was a grade III/VI holosystolic murmur radiating to the left axilla otherwise, head, neck, chest, heart and abdomen exam was unremarkable. Extremities showed no edema. The neurologic exam was normal.

HOSPITAL COURSE: The patient was monitored on the telemetry service and there was no evidence of myocardial infarction. An attempt to perform a treadmill test was made and although the patient was admitted with PVC there was no ST-T wave change, although exercise tolerance was poor. During monitoring on the floor, the patient was noted to have complaints of dizziness and long sinus pauses. This became her current problem and it was clear the patient had developed second-degree AV block. Accordingly, a DDDR pacer was implanted. A Medtronic Elite 7074 SN YE2118171 was placed.

CASE 24

DISCHARGE SUMMARY (cont.)

The patient was asymptomatic after the placement of this and after 2 days of monitoring was discharged. Her only medication was Synthroid 0.1 mg daily. She will be seen in the office in one week and followed by Dr. DeMare for the pacer site.

———————————————
G. Morton, M.D.

GM/LM

Case 24 Study Questions

1. The patient history includes hypercholesterolemia. What is hypercholesterolemia?
2. The patient's history includes a recent PTCA. What does this abbreviation mean?
3. The patient was admitted with PVC. What does this abbreviation mean?
4. During a treadmill test the patient experienced ventricular tachycardia. Look ventricular tachycardia up in your medical dictionary. What was it listed under? What does it mean?
5. One discharge diagnosis is "prolonged sinus pauses." What does this mean?

SECTION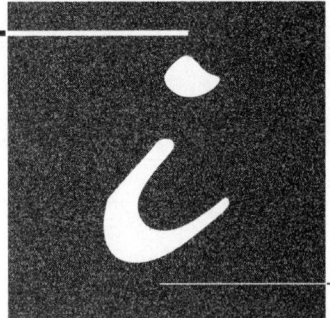

Art for Overhead Transparencies

Overview of Art for Overhead Transparencies

1. Medical Terminology Word Parts
2. Major Body Planes
3. The Skeleton (anterior view)
4. The Skeleton (posterior view)
5. The Skeleton (lateral view)
6. The Skull (anterior view)
7. The Skull (lateral view)
8. Major Muscles (anterior view)
9. Major Muscles (posterior view)
10. The Heart (external view)
11. The Heart (cross section)
12. Systemic and Pulmonary Circulation
13. Structures of the Upper Respiratory Tract
14. Structures of the Bronchial Tree
15. Major Structures of the Digestive System
16. Major Structures of the Urinary System
17. A Nephron Unit and Related Structures
18. The Brain, Spinal Cord and Spinal Nerves (posterior view)
19. The Brain (external lateral view)
20. The Brain (cross section)
21. The Eye (cross section)
22. The Ear (cross section)
23. Structures of the Skin (cross section)
24. Structures of the Endocrine System
25. The Male Pelvis (cross section)
26. The Female Pelvis (cross section)
27. The Developing Fetus (cross section)
28. Examination Positions

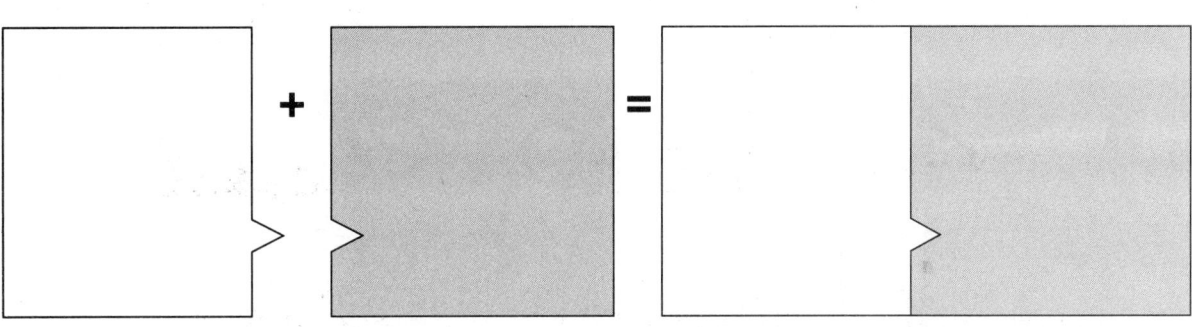

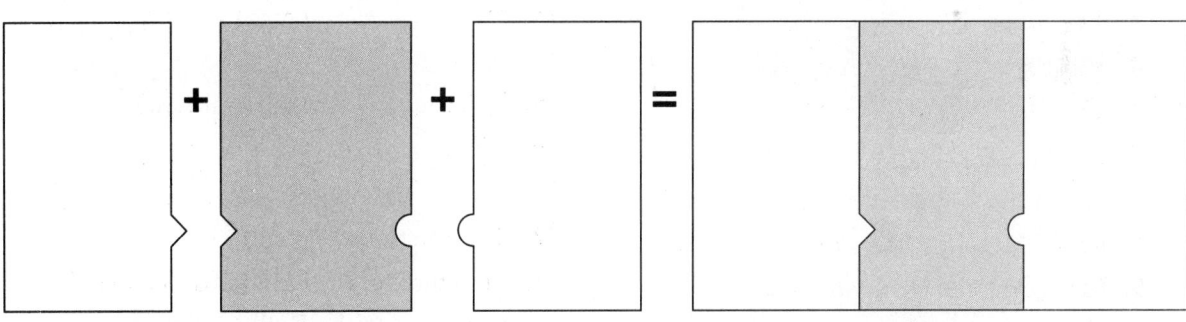

Transparency Master 1 • Medical Terminology Word Parts

216

Overhead Transparencies

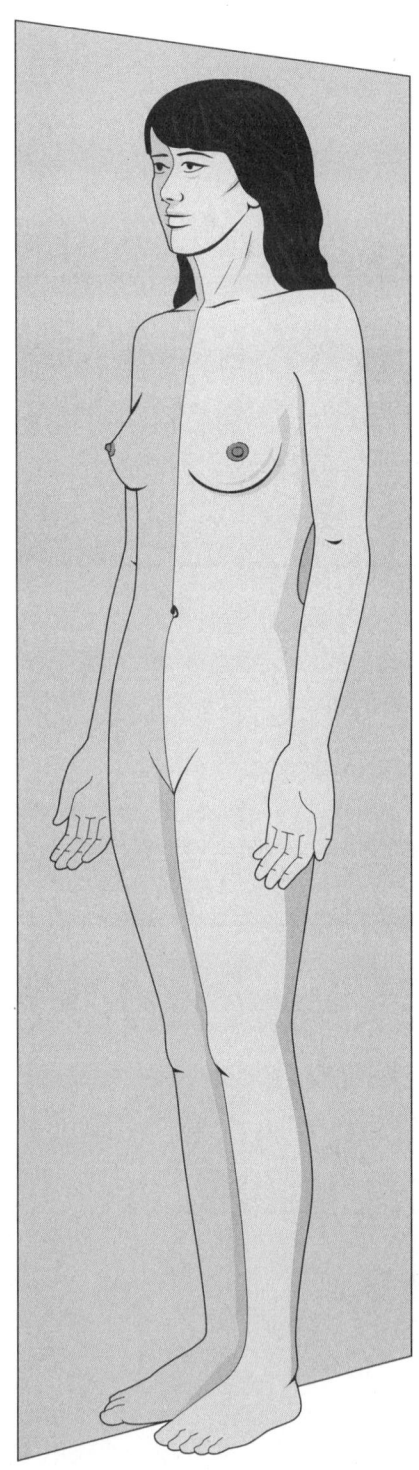
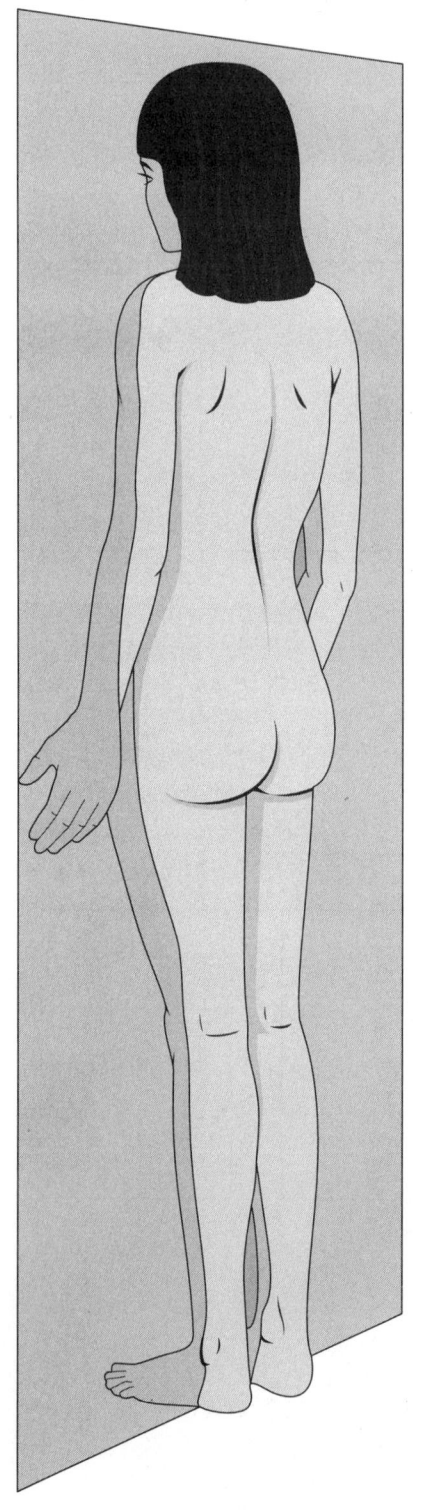

Transparency Master 2 • Major Body Planes

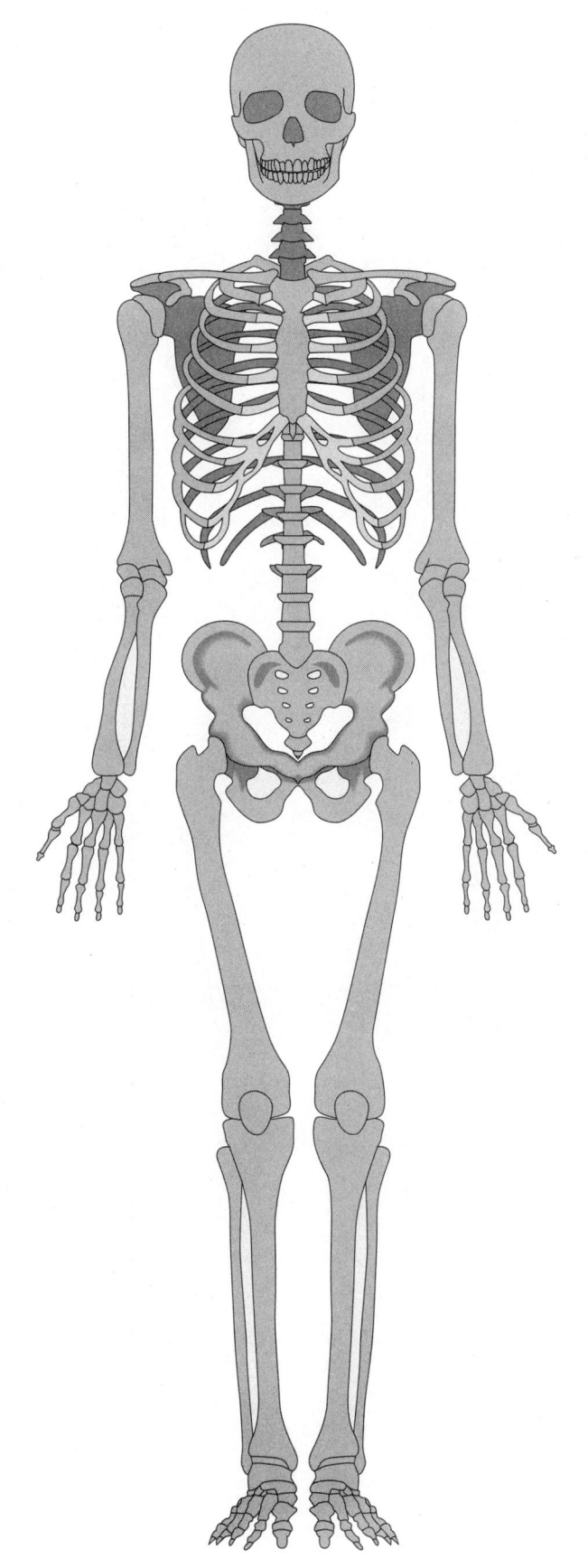

Transparency Master 3 • The Skeleton (anterior view)

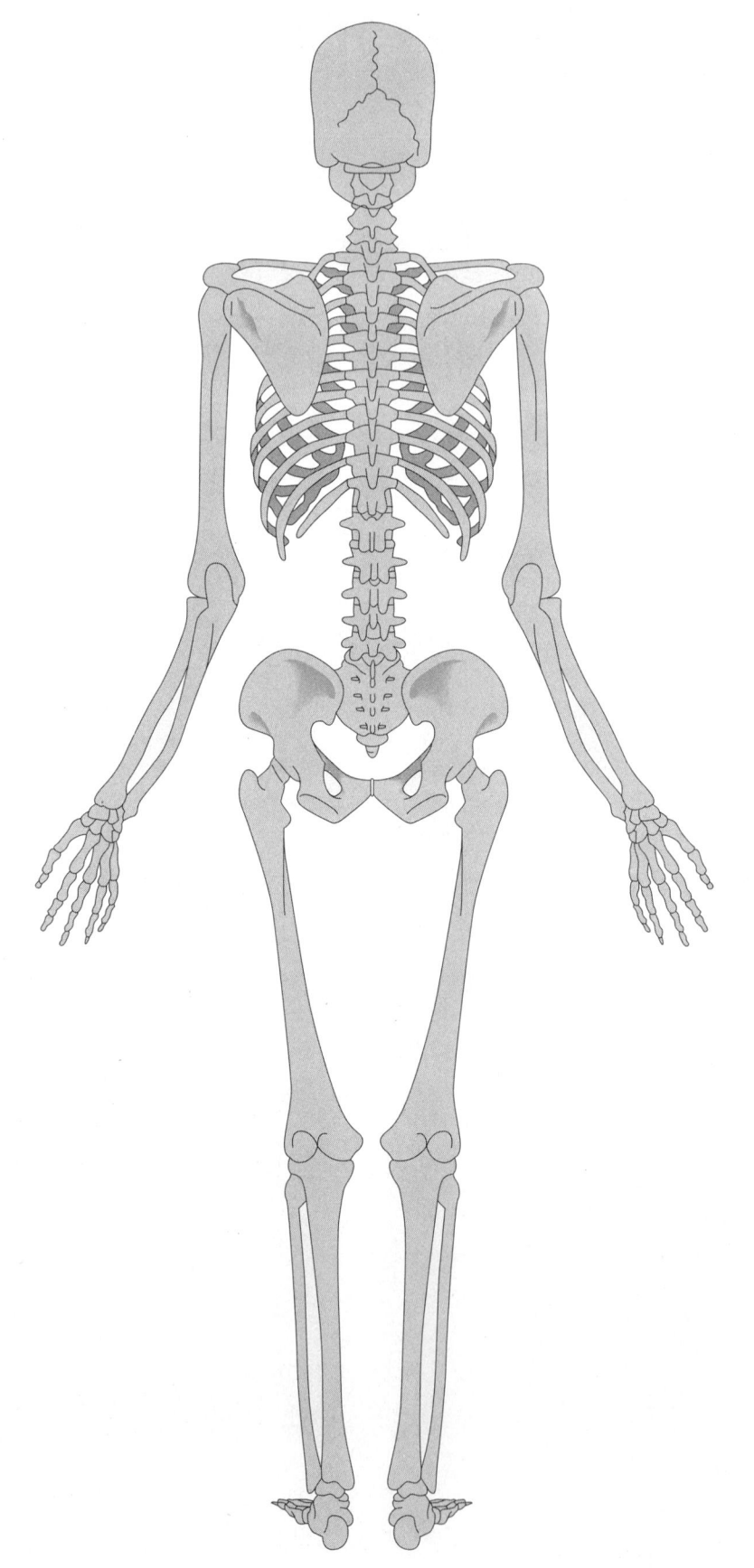

Transparency Master 4 • The Skeleton (posterior view)

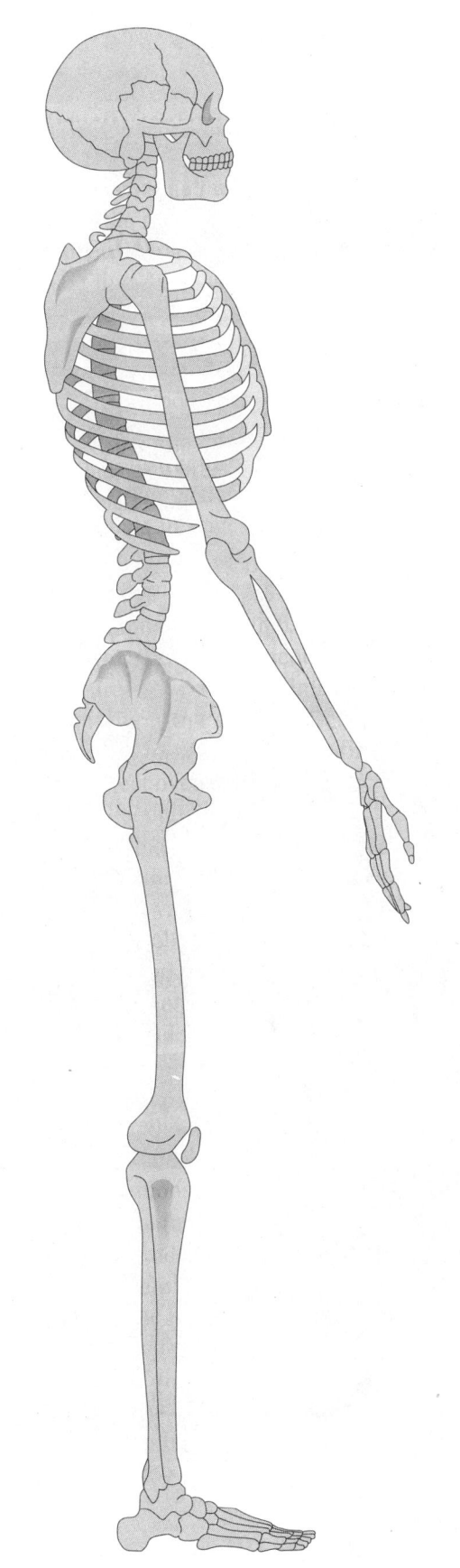

Transparency Master 5 • The Skeleton (lateral view)

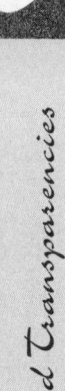

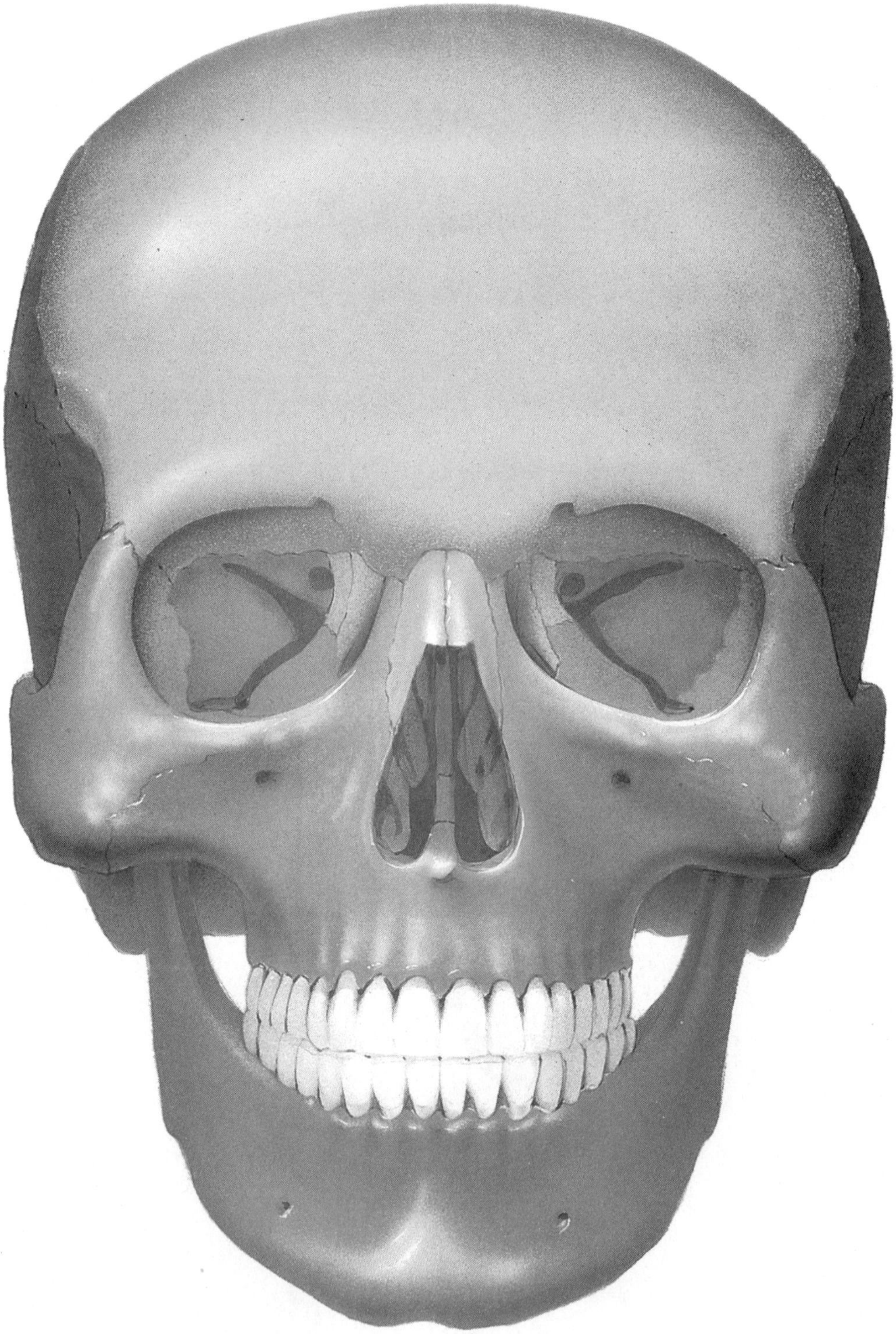

Transparency Master 6 • The Skull (anterior view)

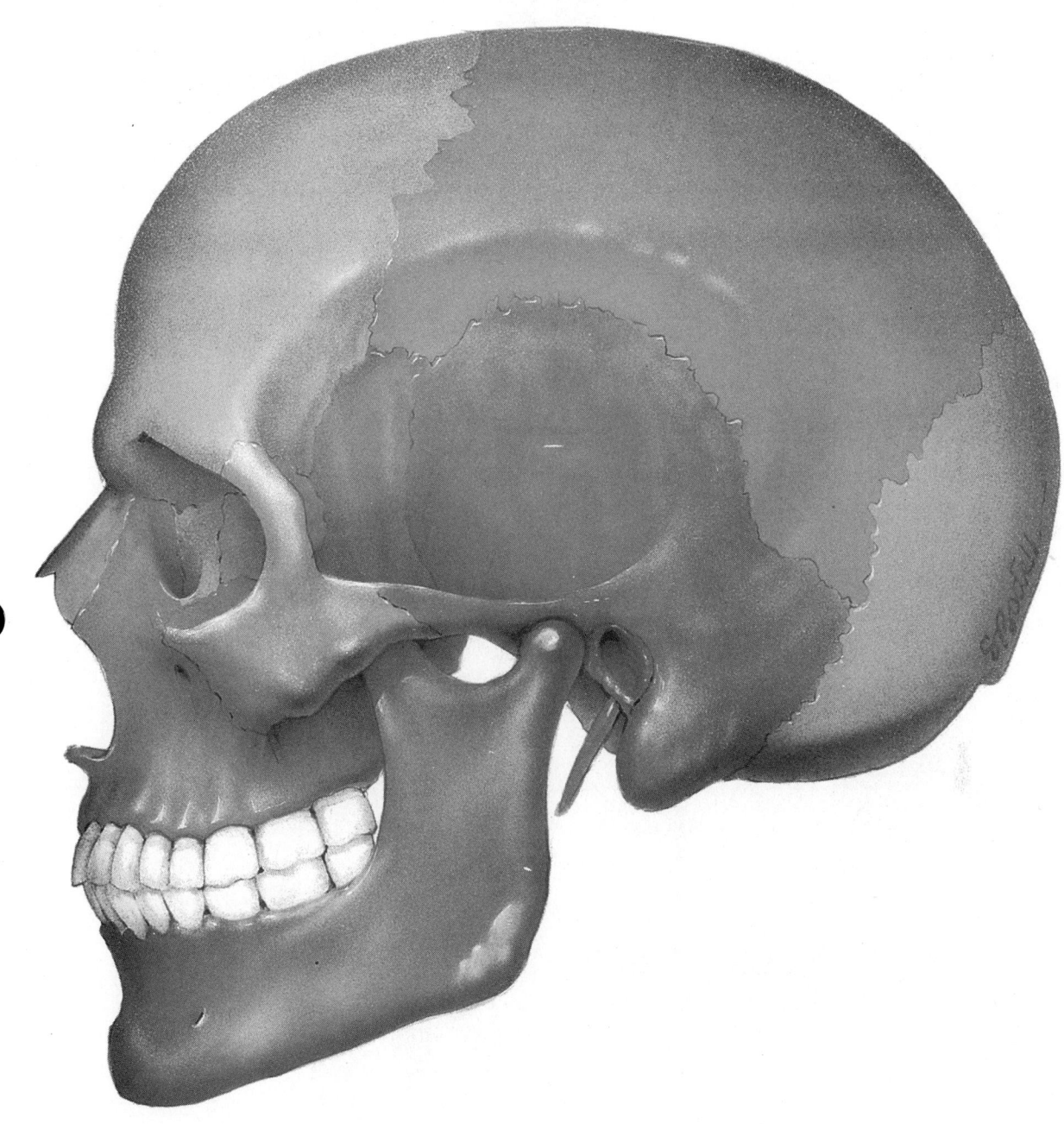

Transparency Master 7 • The Skull (lateral view)

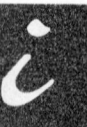

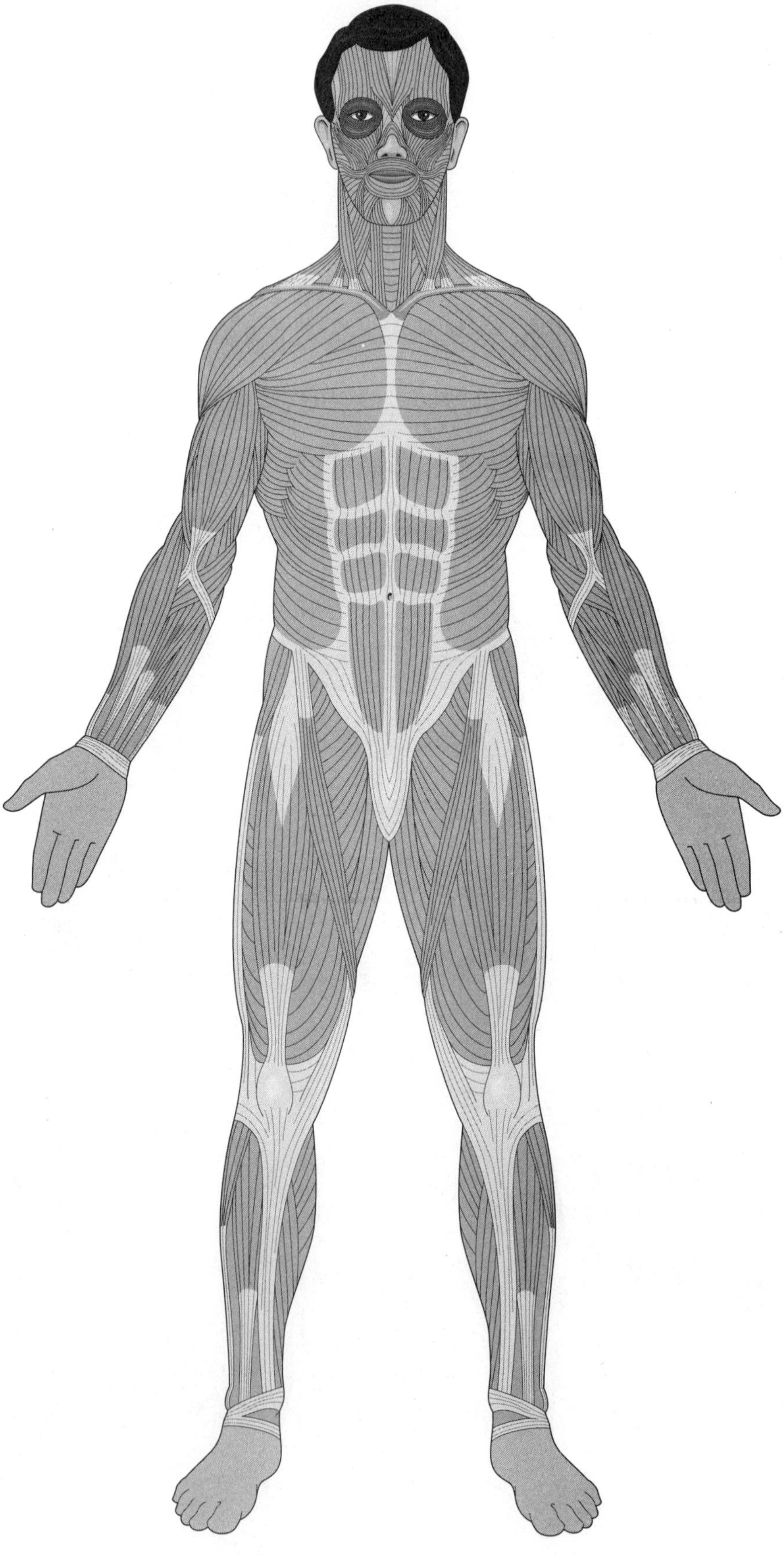

Transparency Master 8 • Major Muscles (anterior view)

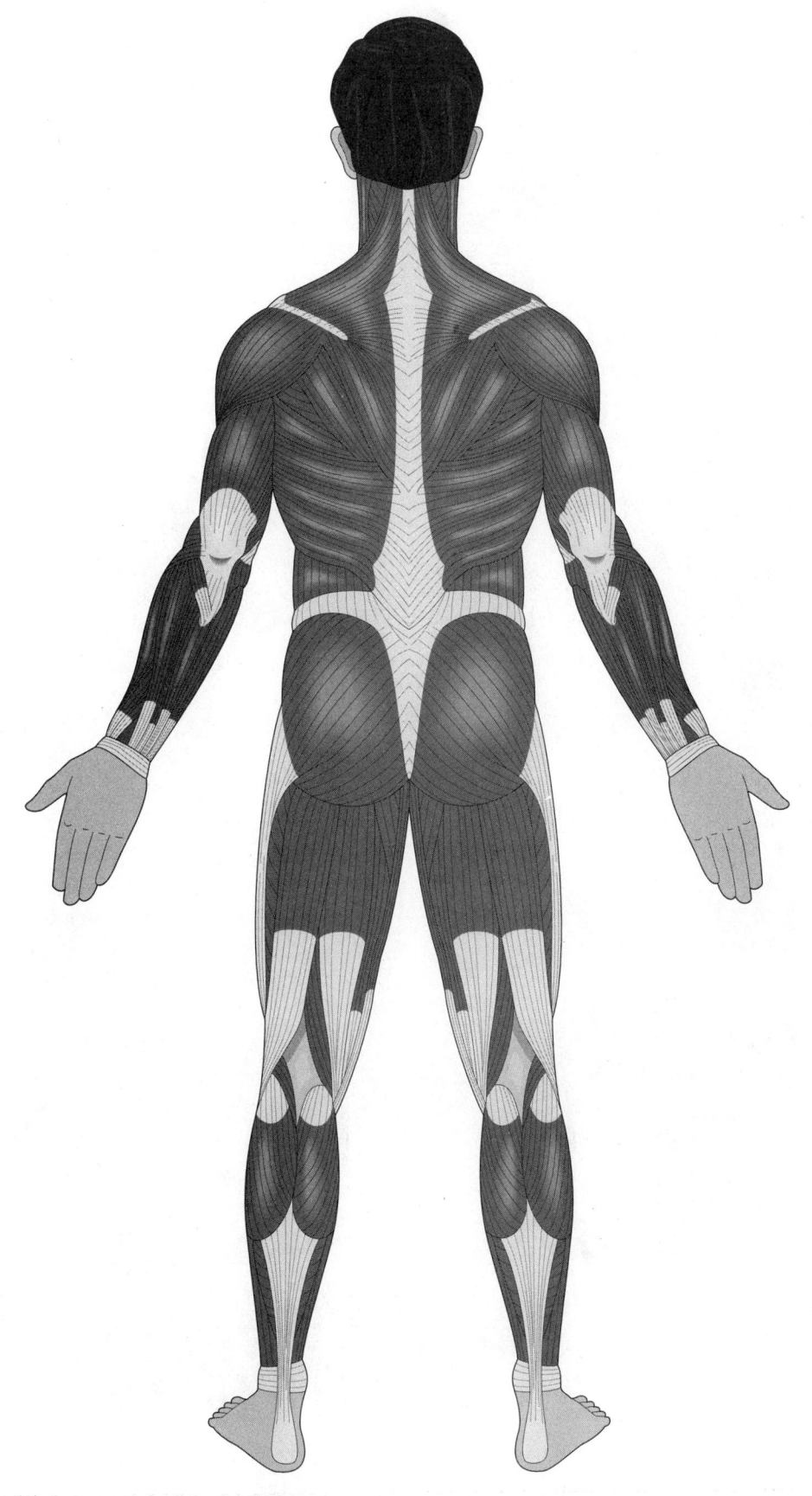

Transparency Master 9 • Major Muscles (posterior view)

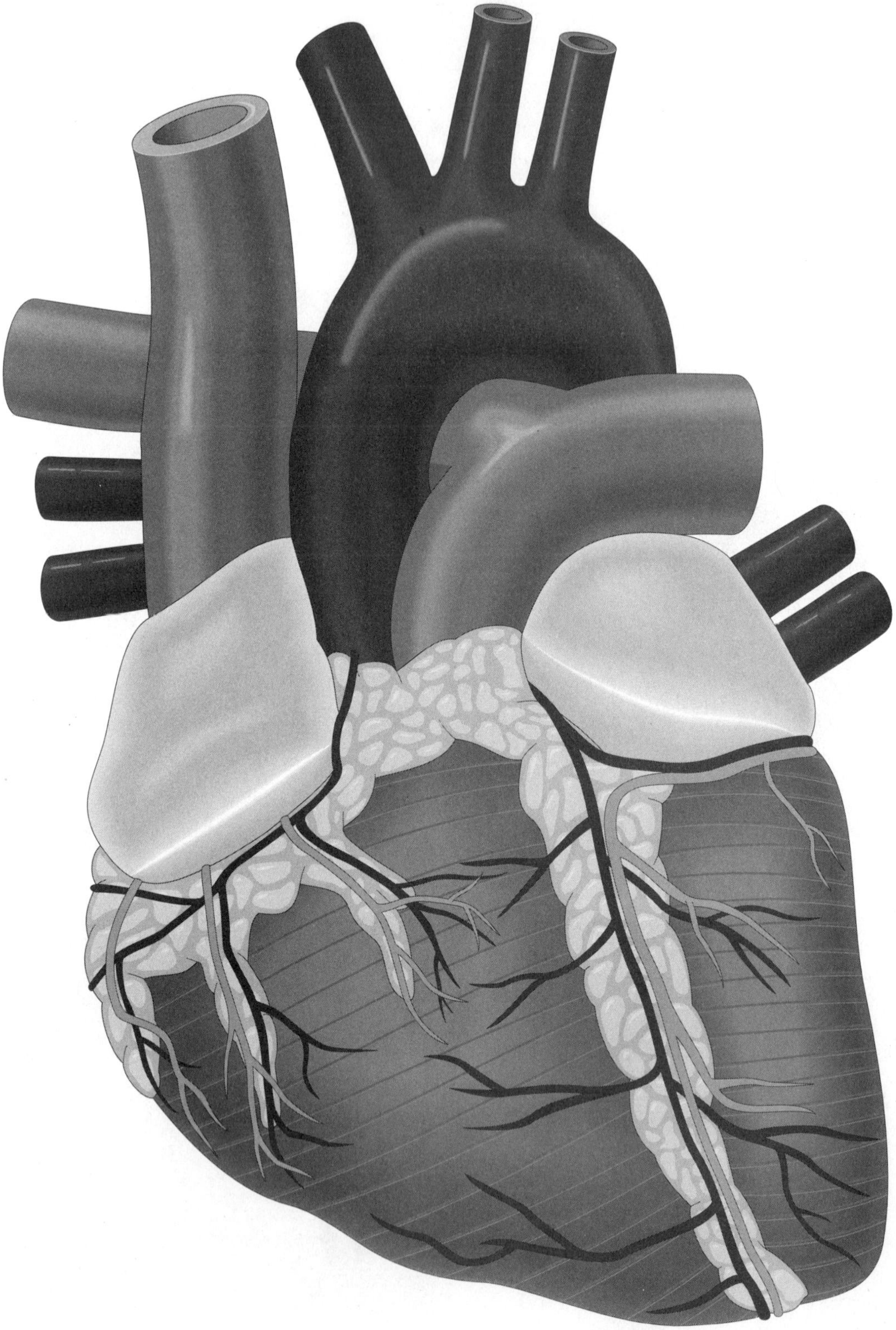

Transparency Master 10 • The Heart (external view)

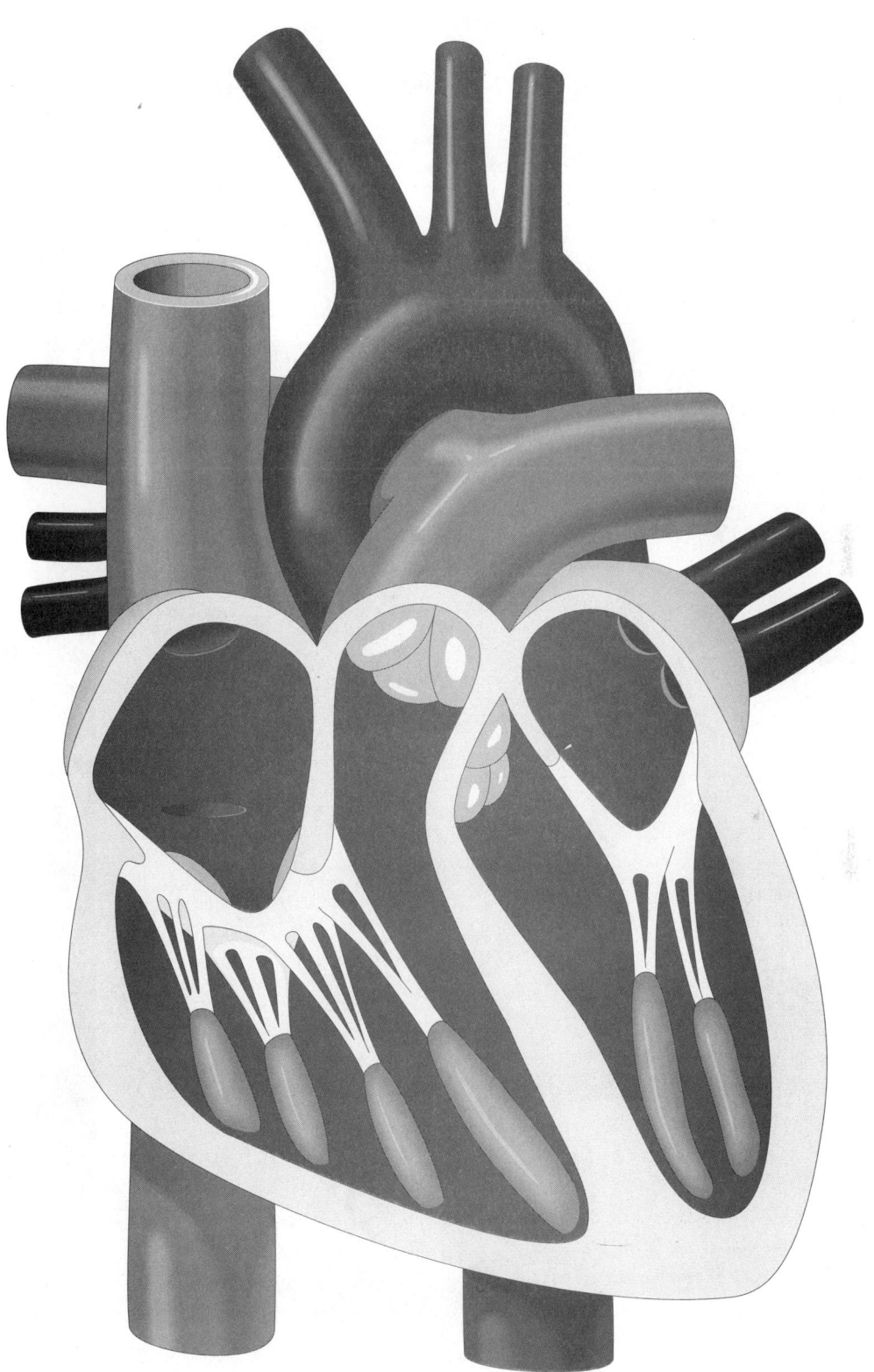

Transparency Master 11 • The Heart (cross section)

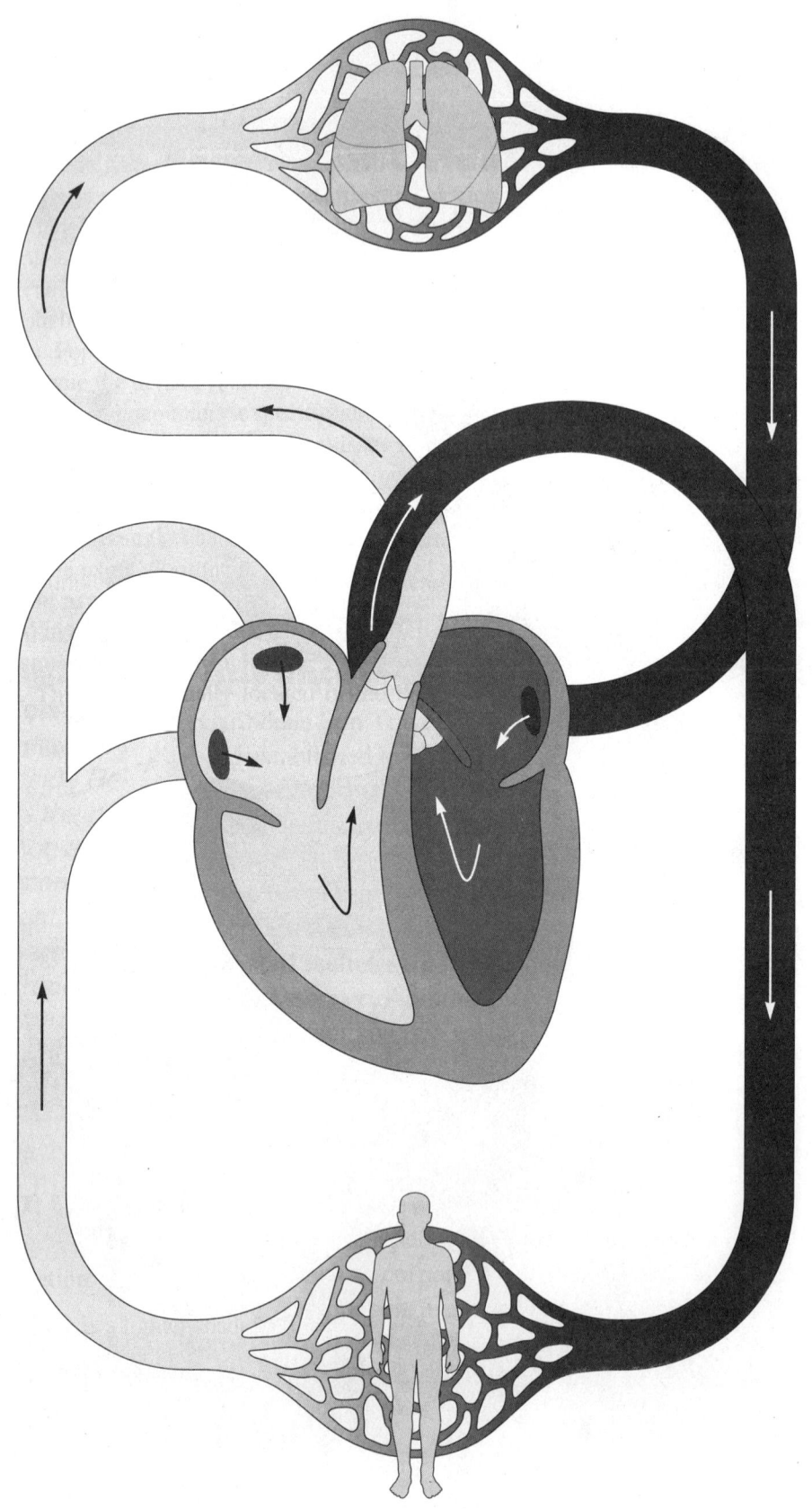

Transparency Master 12 • Systemic and Pulmonary Circulation

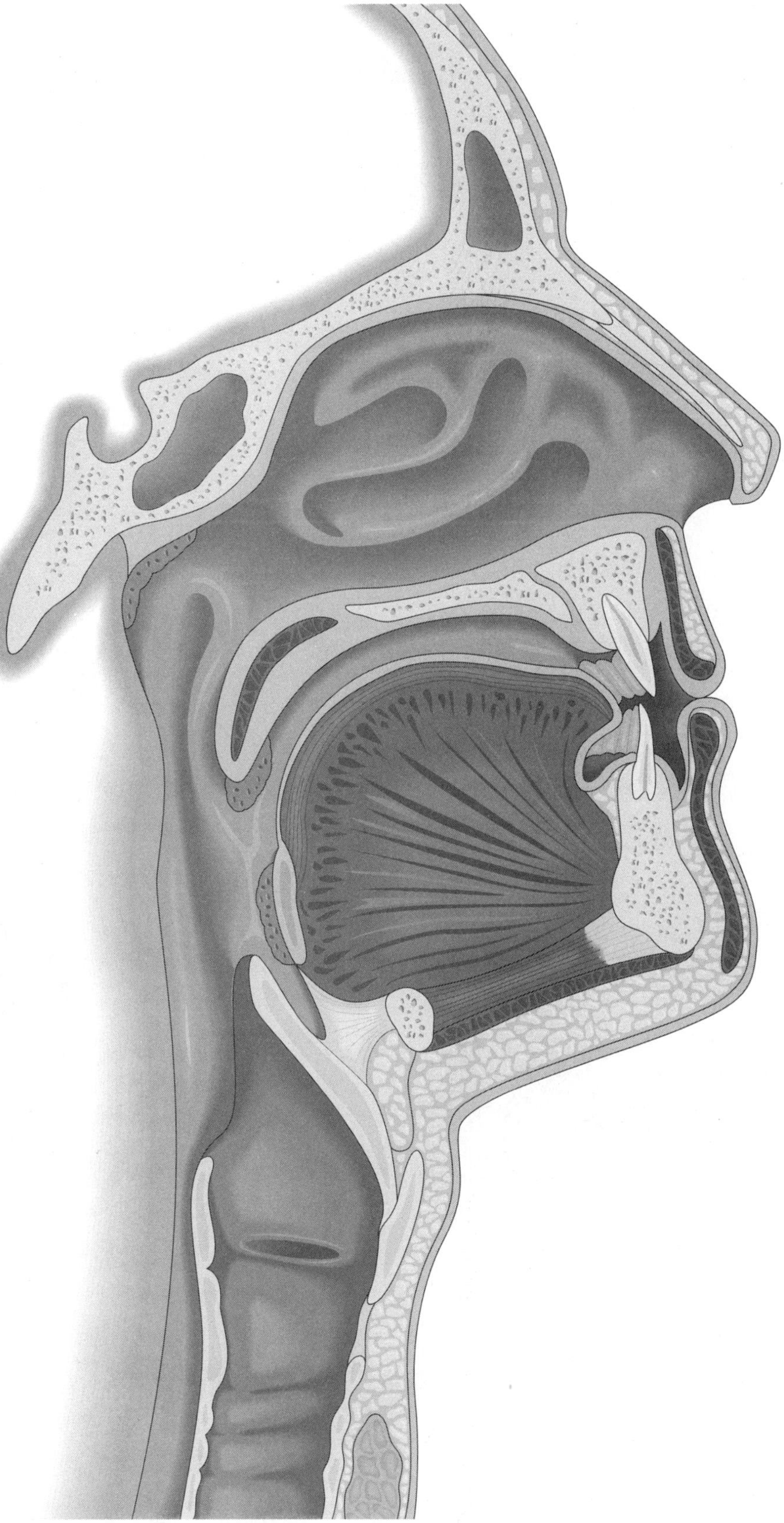

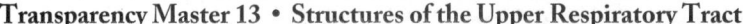

Transparency Master 13 • Structures of the Upper Respiratory Tract

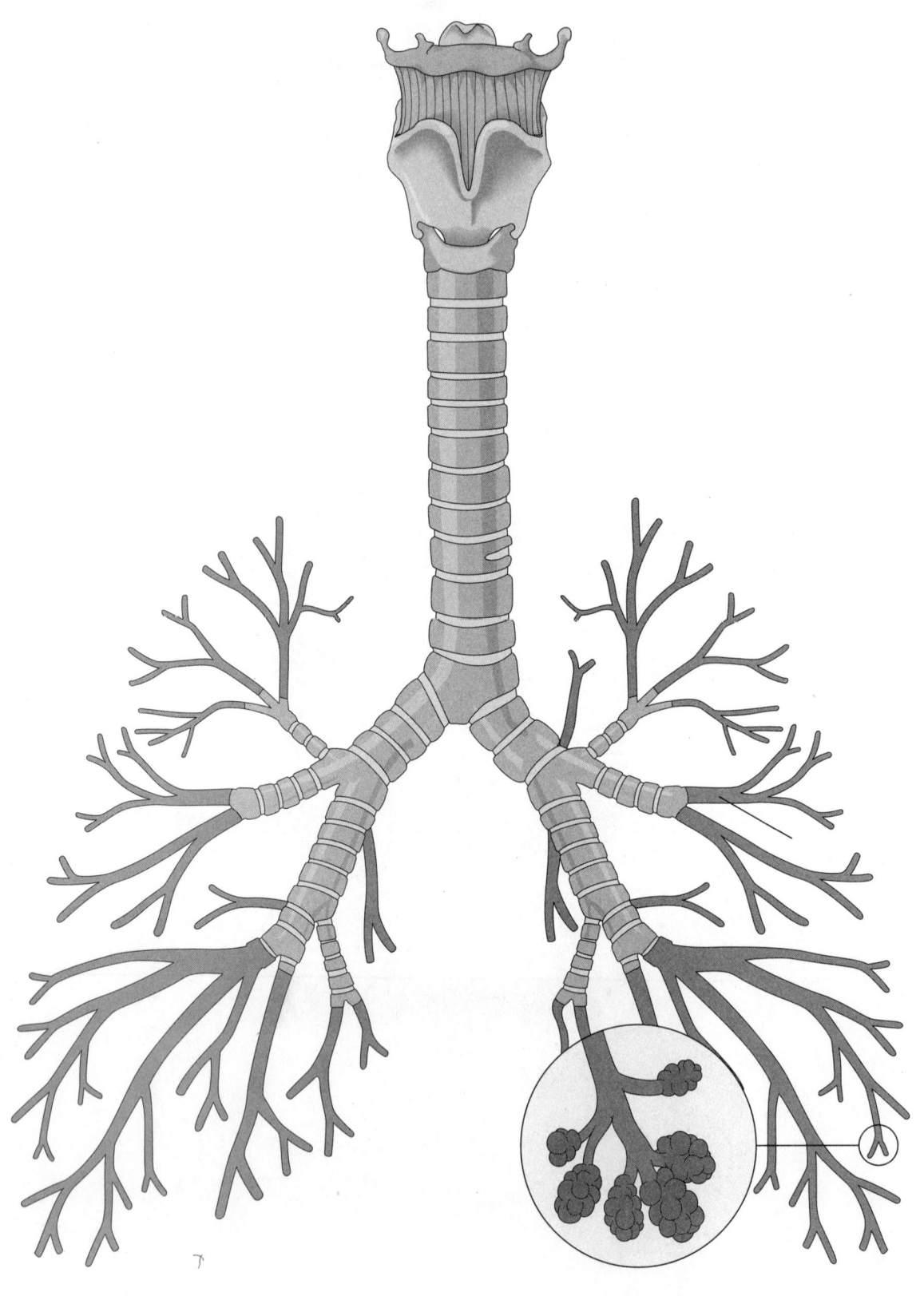

Transparency Master 14 • Structures of the Bronchial Tree

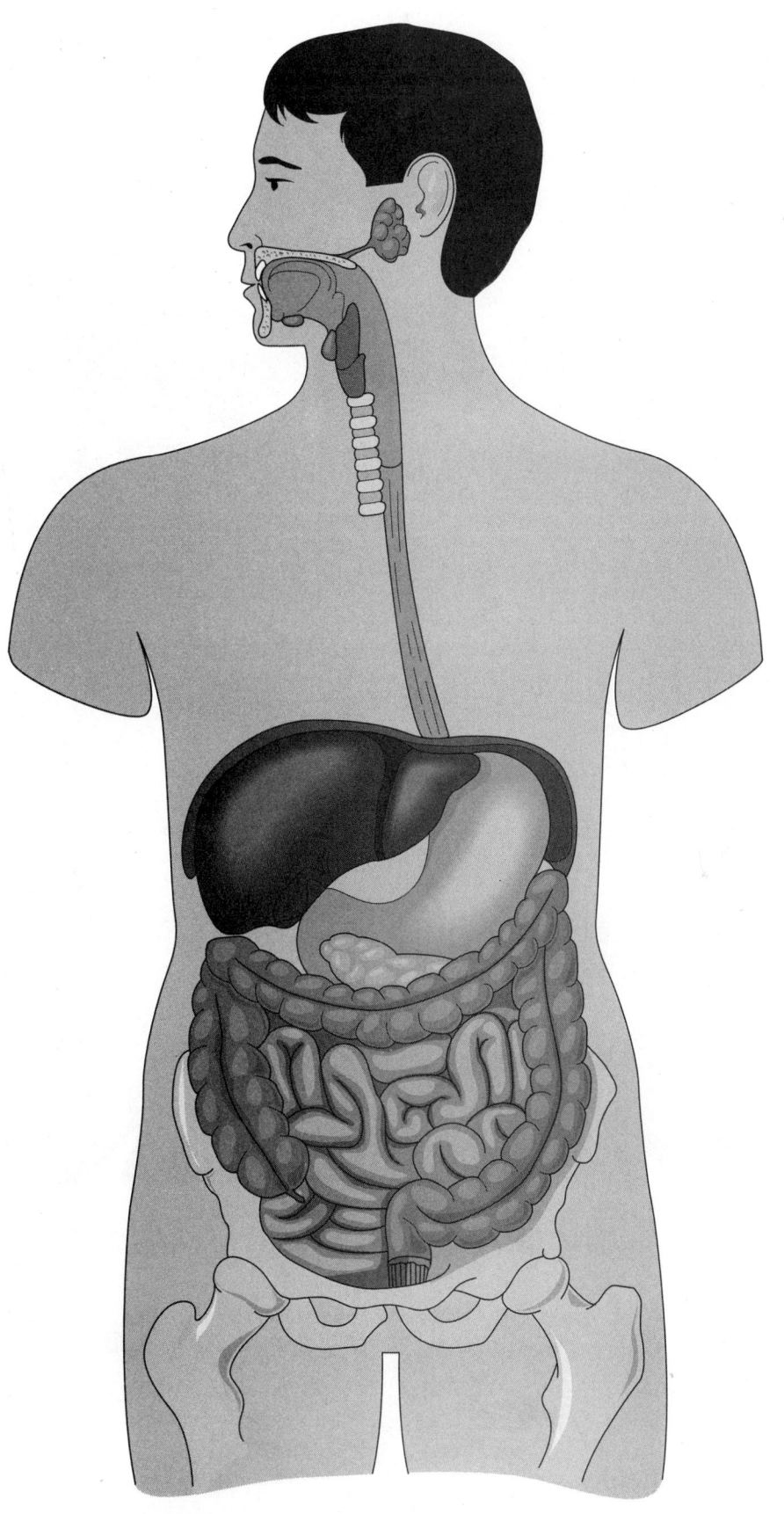

Transparency Master 15 • Major Structures of the Digestive System

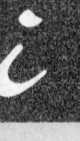

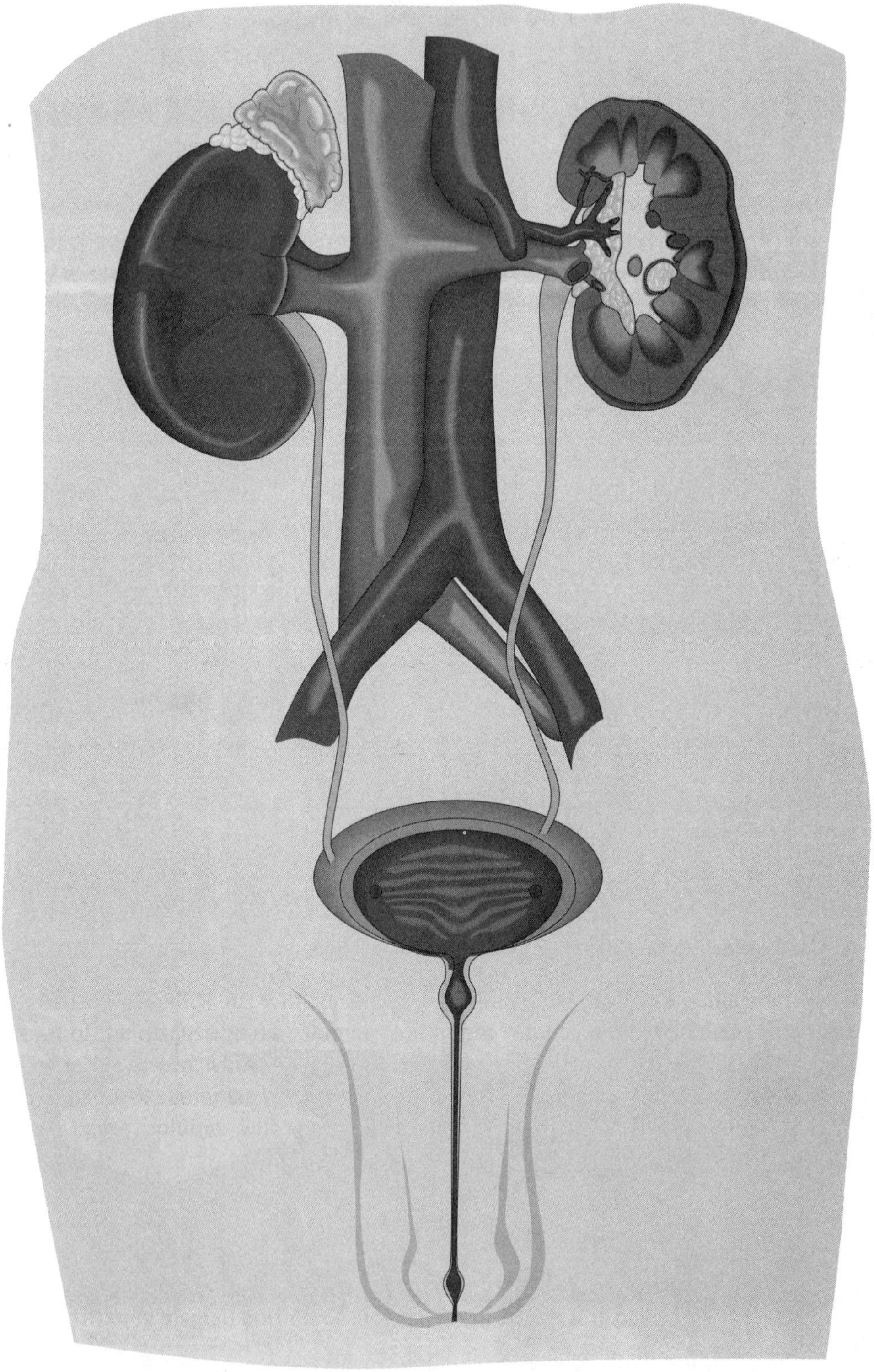

Transparency Master 16 • Major Structures of the Urinary System

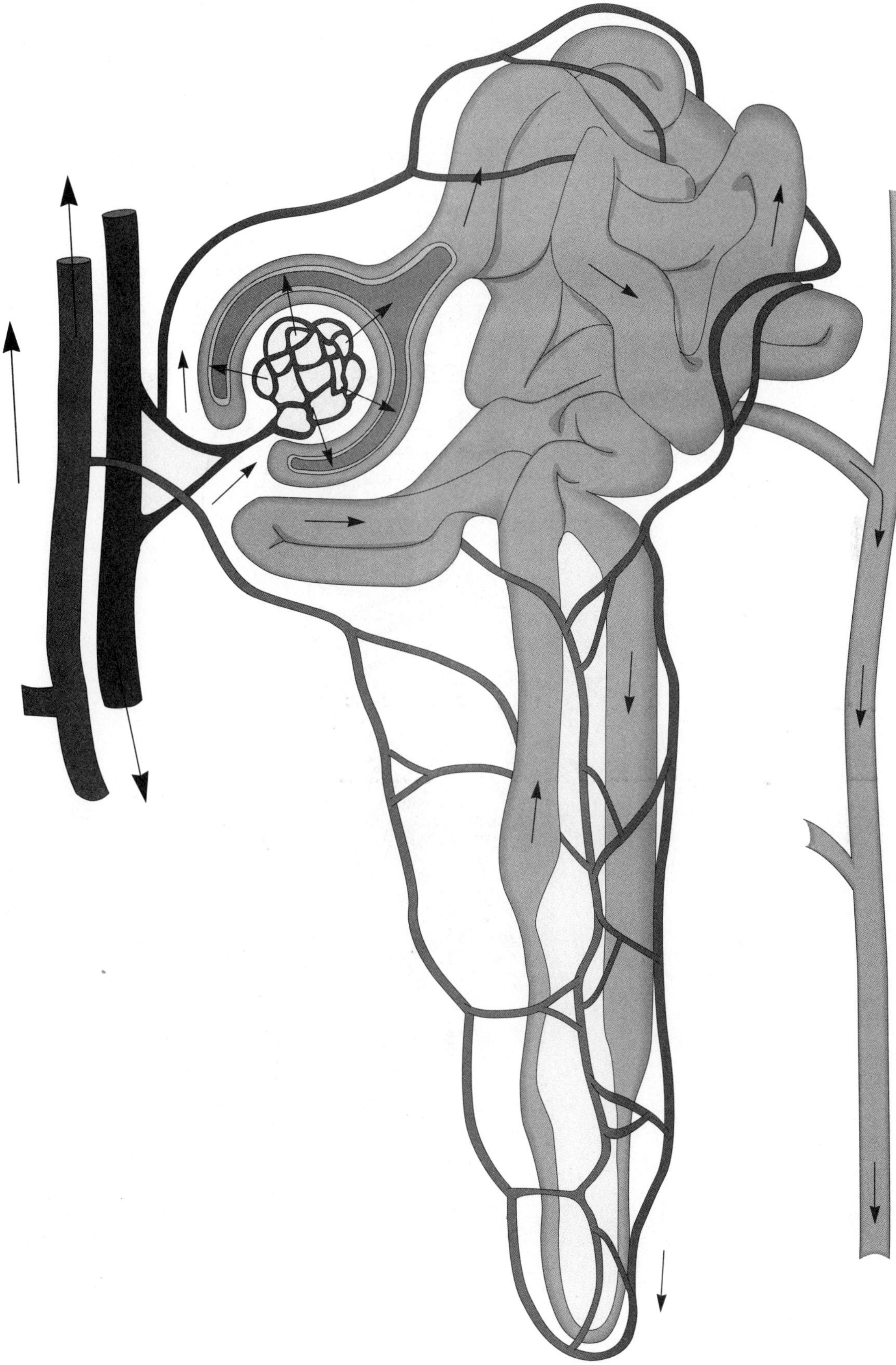

231

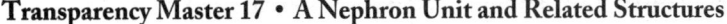

Transparency Master 17 • A Nephron Unit and Related Structures

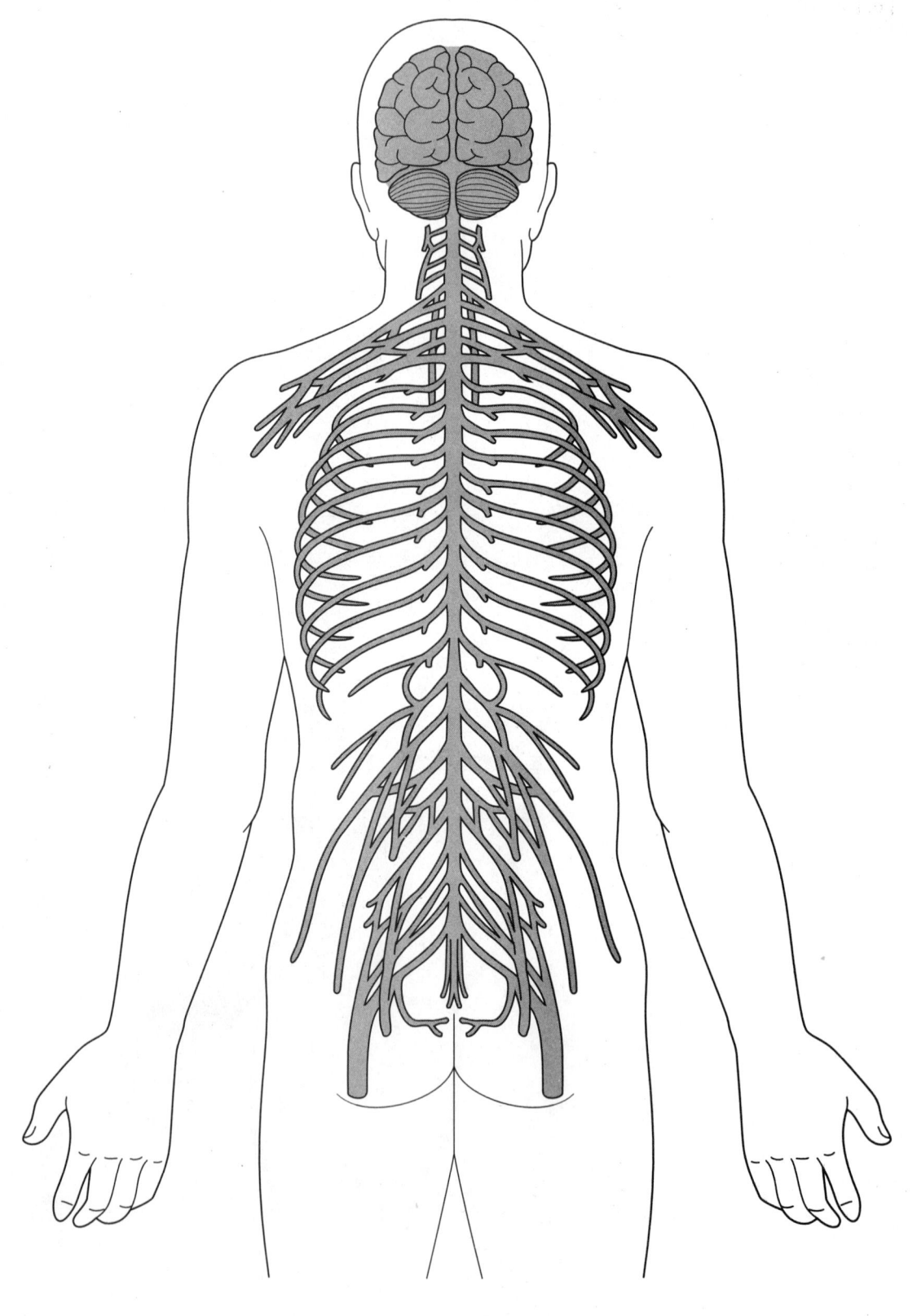

Transparency Master 18 • The Brain, Spinal Cord and Spinal Nerves (posterior view)

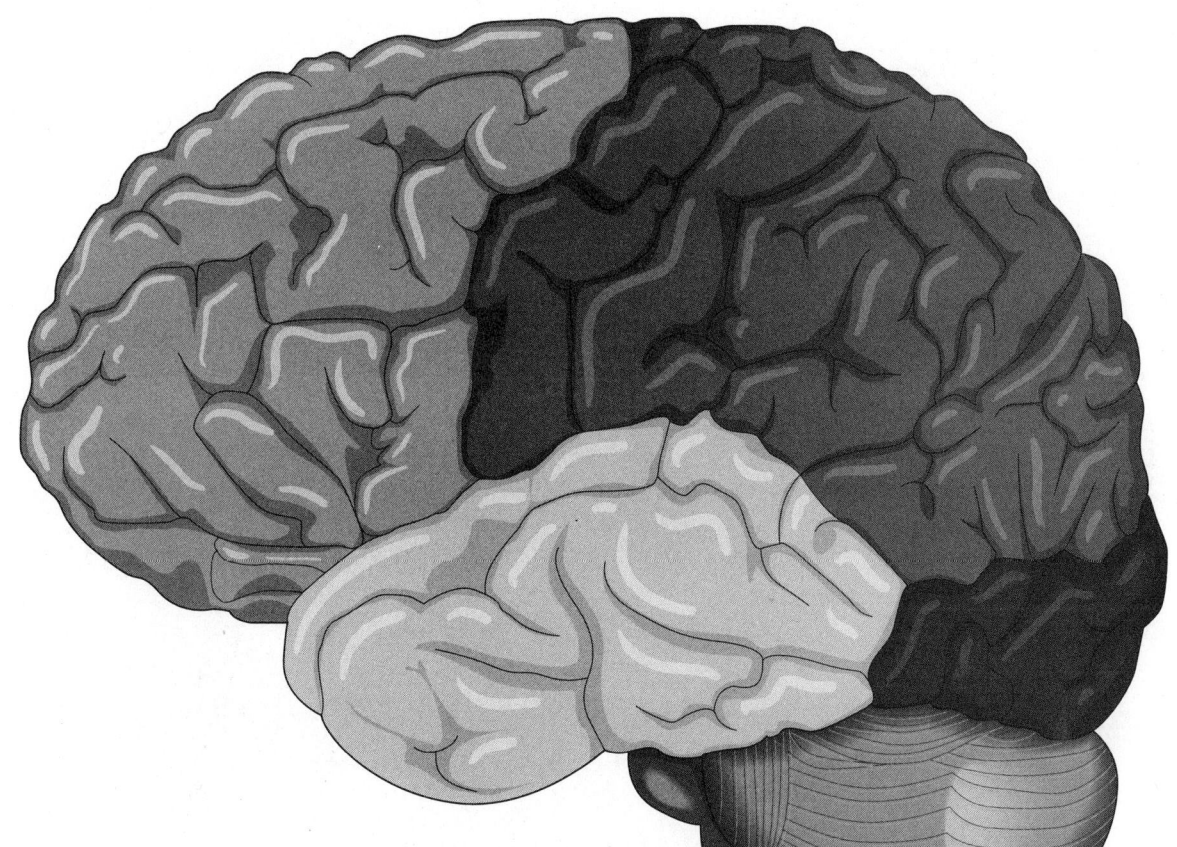

Transparency Master 19 • The Brain (external lateral view)

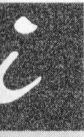

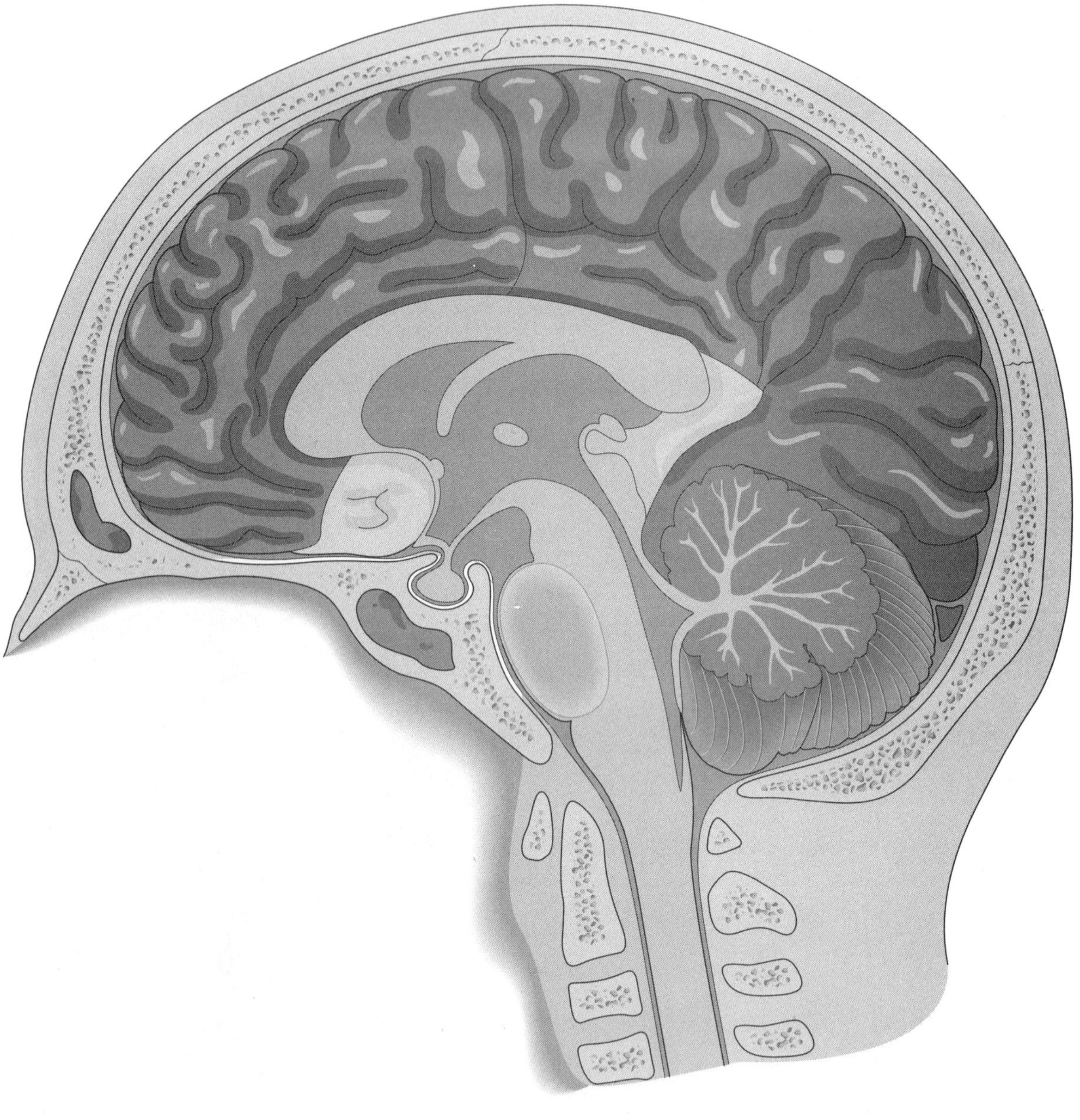

Transparency Master 20 • The Brain (cross section)

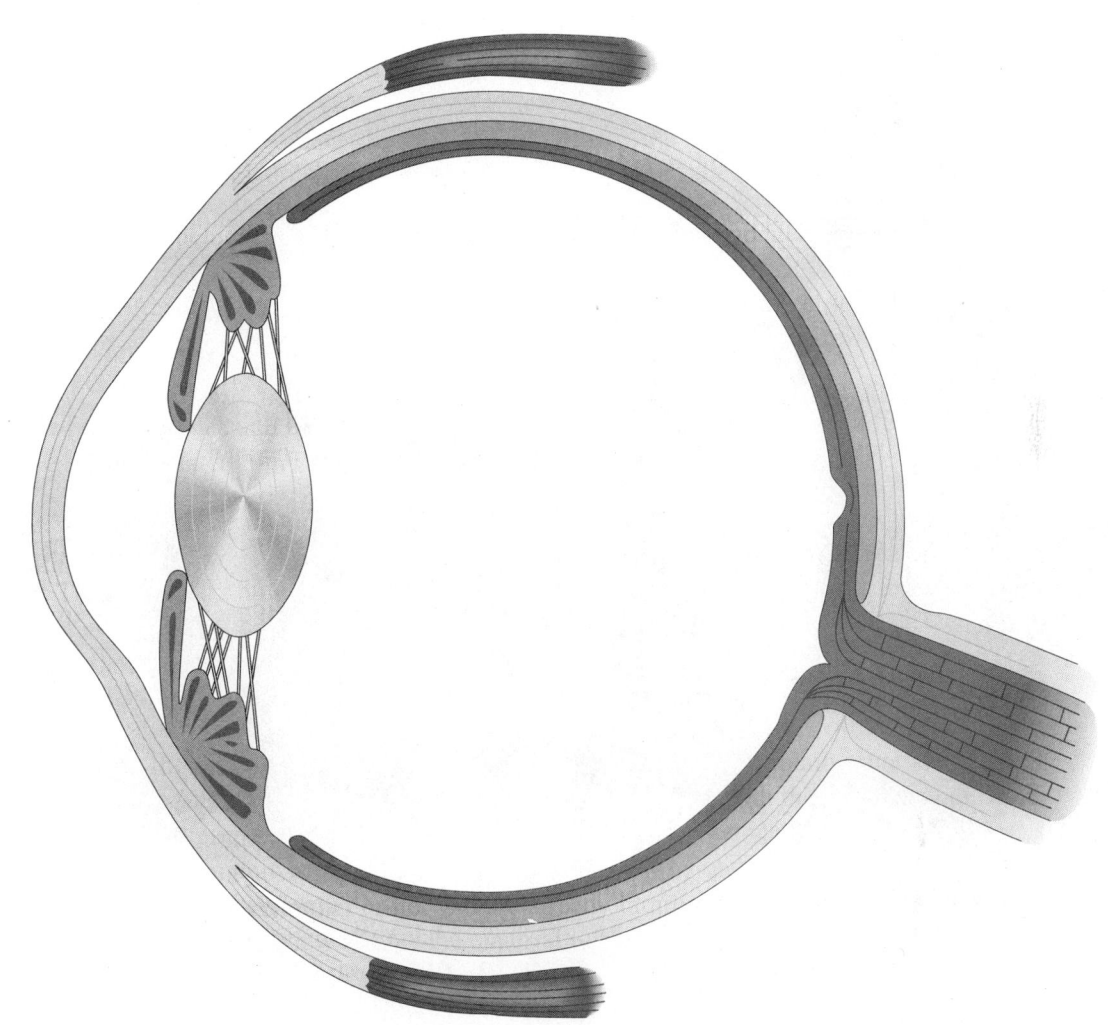

Transparency Master 21 • The Eye (cross section)

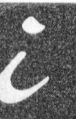

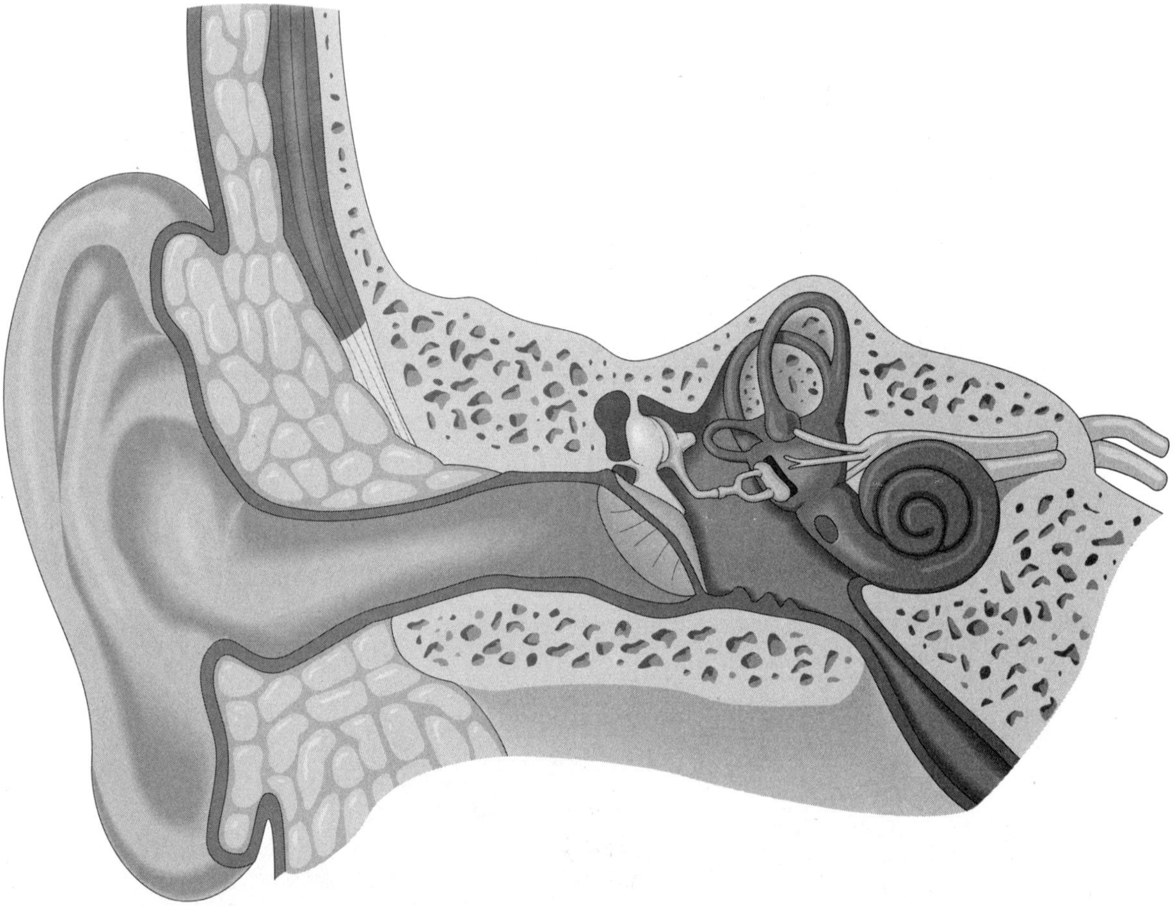

Transparency Master 22 • The Ear (cross section)

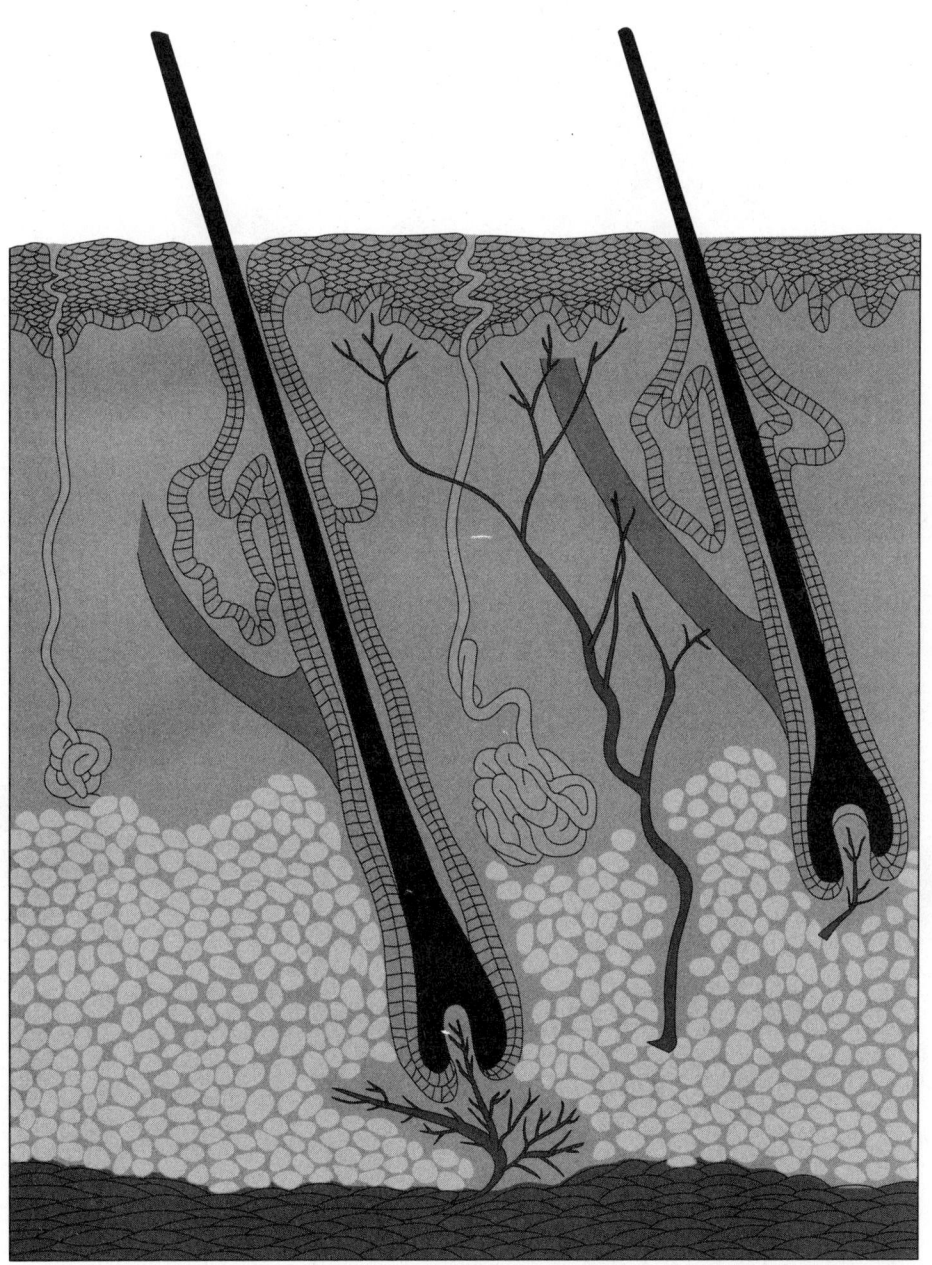

Transparency Master 23 • Structures of the Skin (cross section)

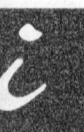

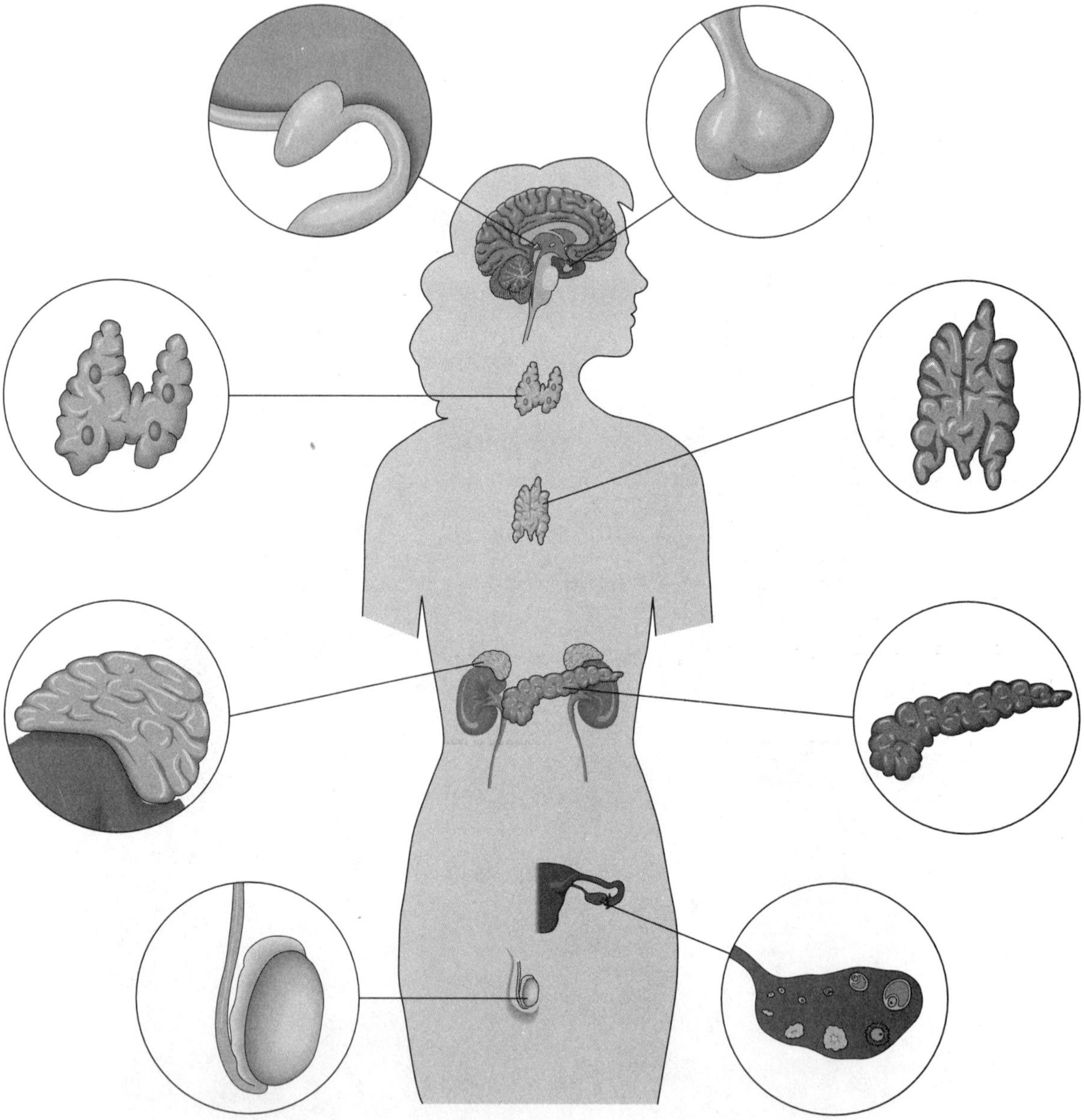

Transparency Master 24 • Structures of the Endocrine System

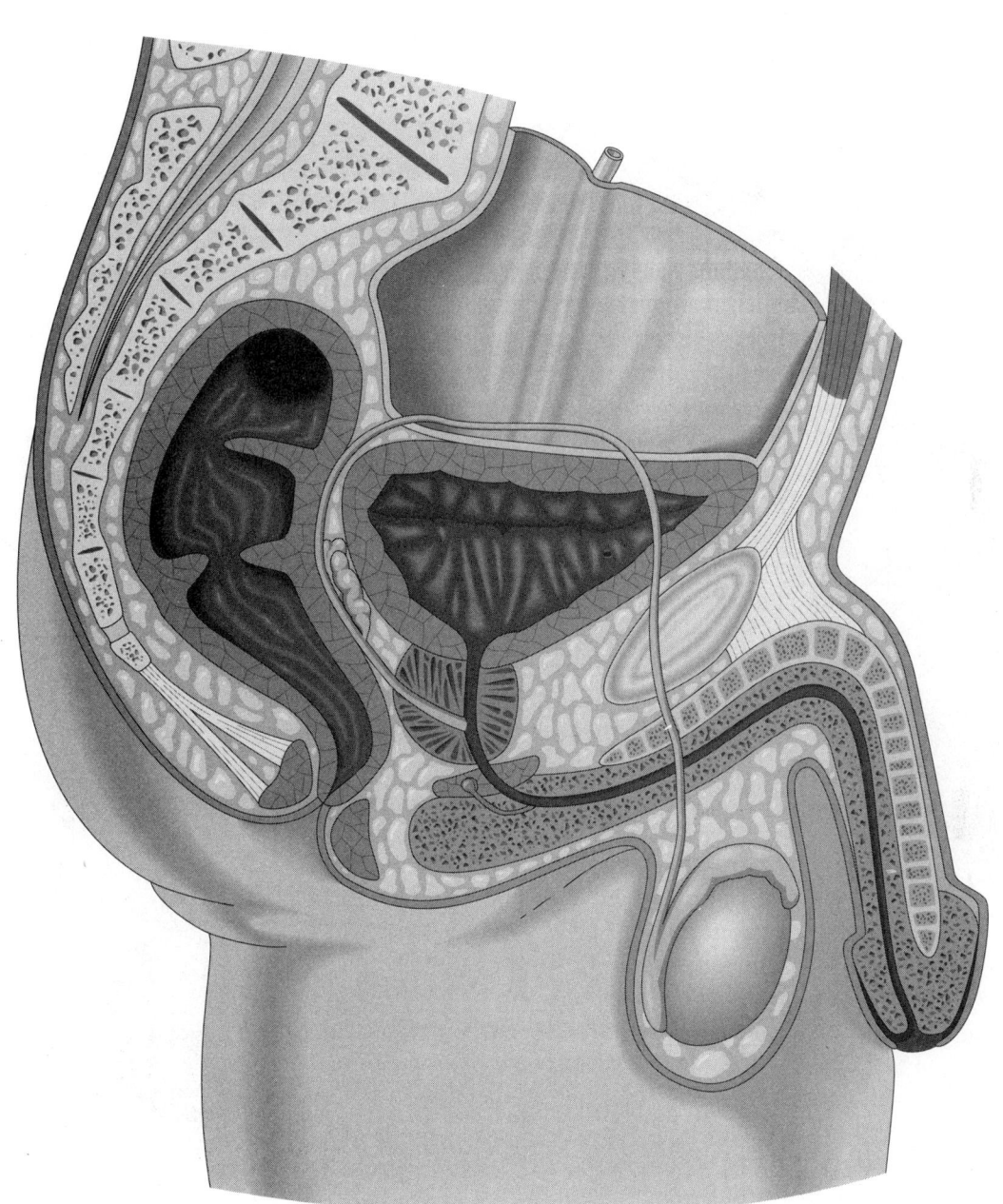

Transparency Master 25 • The Male Pelvis (cross section)

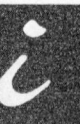

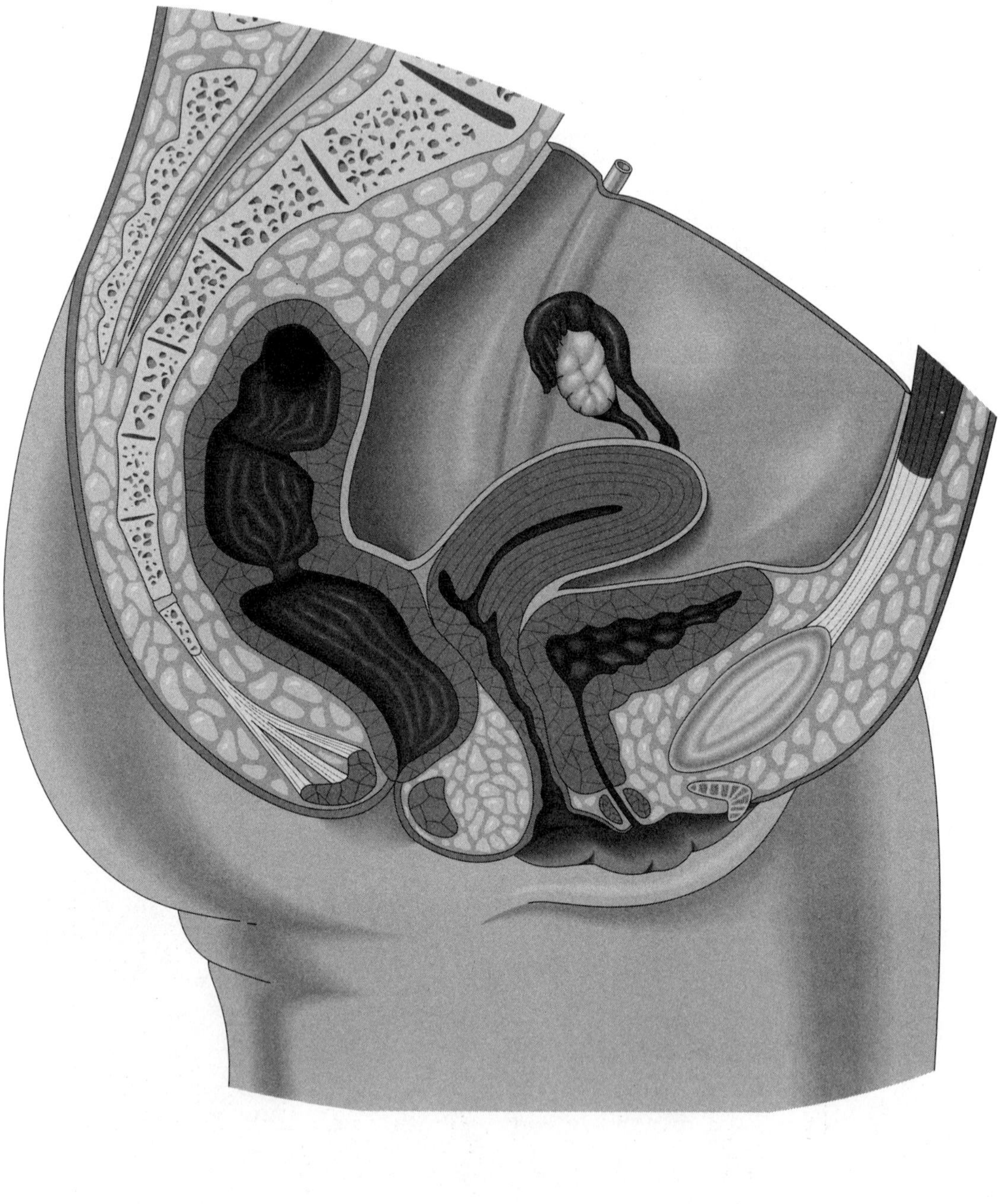

Transparency Master 26 • The Female Pelvis (cross section)

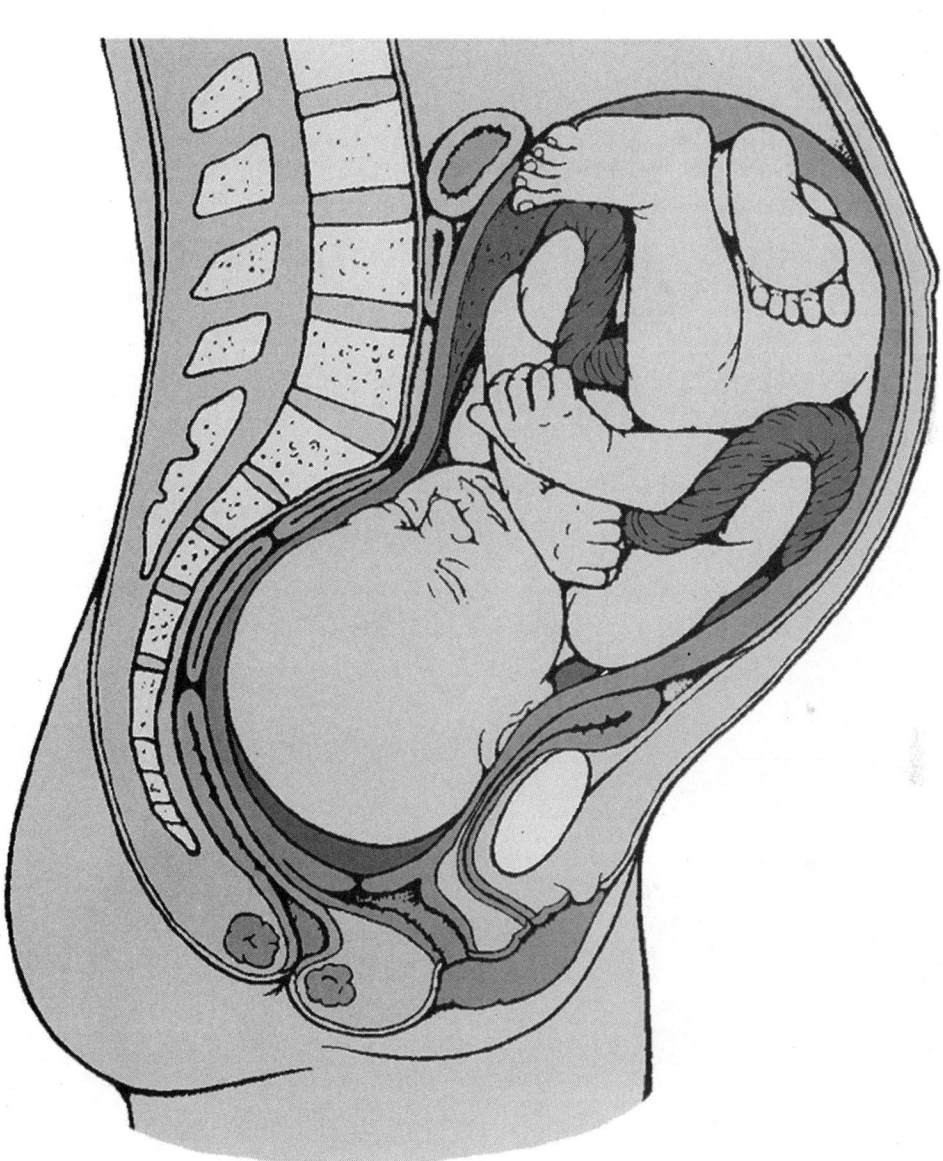

Transparency Master 27 • The Developing Fetus (cross section)

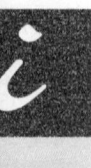

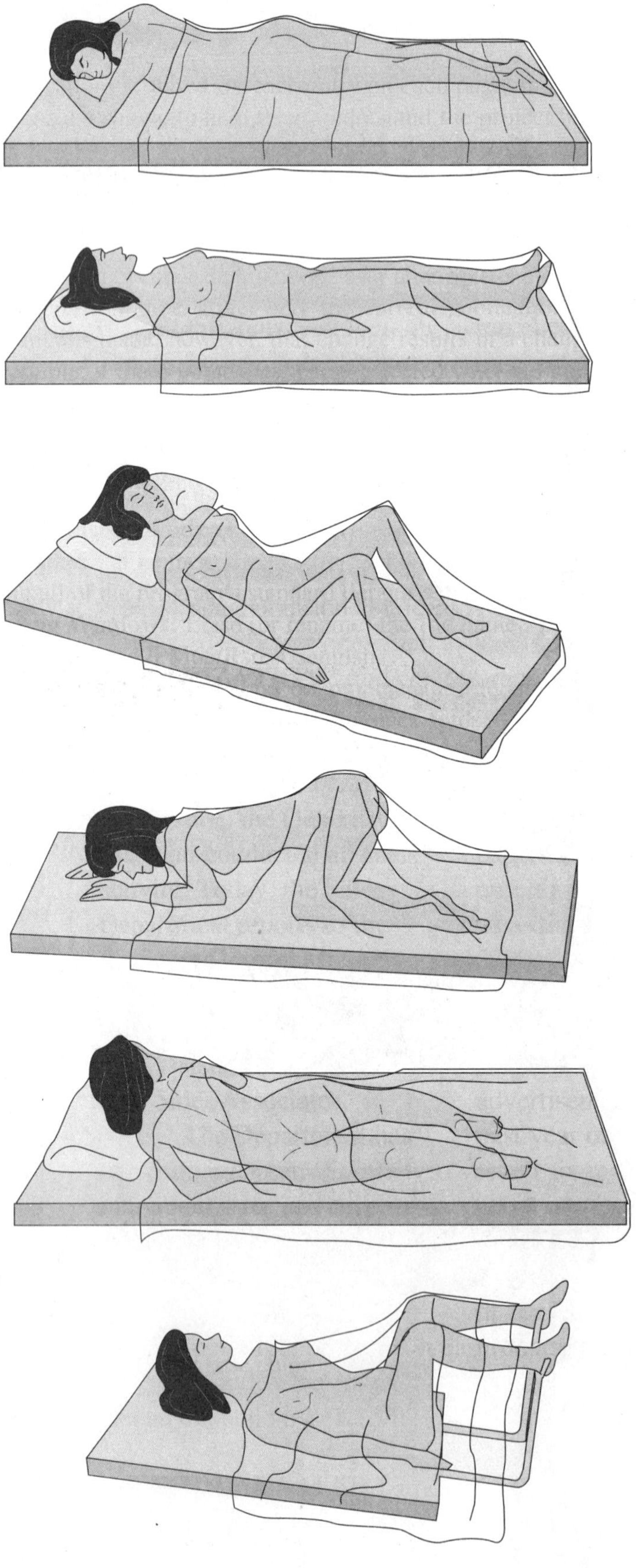

Transparency Master 28 • Examination Positions